Intrinsic mutagenesis:
A genetic approach to ageing

Intrinsic mutagenesis: A genetic approach to ageing

Sir Macfarlane Burnet

A WILEY BIOMEDICAL-HEALTH PUBLICATION

JOHN WILEY & SONS
New York · Toronto

Published in the USA and Canada
by John Wiley & Sons Inc., New York

First published in the United Kingdom by
MTP
Medical and Technical Publishing Co. Ltd.,
Lancaster, England.

ISBN-13: 978-94-011-6608-9 e-ISBN-13: 978-94-011-6606-5
DOI: 10.1007/978-94-011-6606-5

Library of Congress Catalog Card No. 74-6978

Contents

INTRODUCTION

This book is something which almost accidentally has developed very differently from how it was initially planned. The intention was to elaborate the part played by the immune system in ageing with the role of the thymus as central theme. It was to be essentially an expansion of a lecture I gave in 1970 and would inevitably have been concerned with much the same material as Walford's book, *The Immunologic Theory of Aging*, though from a different slant.

What changed its character arose from a series of attempts to find logical connection between two findings that most gerontologists regard as axiomatic: that the lifespan of a mammal is genetically determined, and that the actual process of ageing is an accumulation of genetic error, of somatic mutations. It is possible that the connection is so indirect, circuitous and multiform that generations of detailed and unattractive research will be needed to elucidate it, or, more likely, the whole matter discarded as a non-problem. But a more inspiring approach does seem possible. The working hypothesis, which halfway through its writing became the new central theme of the book, arose when I was a member of a committee appointed by the Australian Academy of Science at the request of the Australian Government to advise on the danger from French nuclear tests in the South Pacific. As every radiobiologist knows, the problem of whether increments of ionizing radiation well below the level of background radiation have any significantly damaging biological effect is insoluble scientifically. There is a reasonable way of using a certain rule to calculate what might be the upper limit of any effect, but beyond that we can only say that it is something less than this, and it may be zero. The assignment made me specially interested in the topic of DNA repair. I had known that something of the sort was possible in bacteria, but had never realized how elaborate a battery of enzymes was concerned with monitoring, excision, and repair of DNA in *E. coli*, and by every analogy in all mammalian cells. The hypothesis of intrinsic mutagenesis arose from mulling over the significance of that elaborate repair system.

In brief, the hypothesis ascribes mutation wholly to error production by the enzymatic machinery responsible for DNA duplication and repair. The established effect of the conventional physical and chemical mutagens is regarded as due simply to enlarged opportunity of error proportional to the amount of DNA repair required. I am very much aware that to deny any direct mutagenic action by environmental impact is likely to be regarded as a contorted approach to a phenomenon that other people regard as something well established and readily understood. It will be categorically opposed by many as an attempt to play down the hazards of the military, industrial and medical uses of ionizing radiation. A more legitimate objection is to ask whether the suggested approach has implications which are susceptible to experimental test. The extreme complexity of the genetic mechanism is becoming more and more evident, and it could well eventuate that a precise molecular understanding of mutagenesis will stay forever beyond the reach of experiment. I am more hopeful, and the main claim I would make and the best justification for writing this book is that the hypothesis calls for the application of already available techniques of molecular genetics to a wide range of problems in the physiology and pathology of old age.

The real difficulty in writing this book has been to provide an account of what is basically a rather simple concept for people interested in biology generally, but more particularly biology as it applies to human affairs, and at the same time provide adequate evidence from the experimental literature to justify the point of view adopted to those professionally interested in mutagenesis. I find the solution I have adopted rather unsatisfactory, but, given the current situation of academic biology, I cannot devise a better one. I have had a wide experience in most of the biological sciences that impinge upon medicine and a special interest in the application of Darwinian principles to the phenomena of disease and the interactions of cells within the body. The concept of intrinsic mutagenesis is, I believe, a logical extension of Darwinism, just as the clonal selection theory of antibody production was. Unfortunately, if the concept is valid, it covers the whole of biology, and the days when Darwin could apply his concept of natural selection to almost literally everything in current biological knowledge are long past. It is completely impossible nowadays to attempt a full scale discussion at technical level of any topic that covers more than one specialized field. All that I have been able to attempt is to present the general concept with such explanatory or illustrative material from fields of my own interest as seemed likely to help make its significance clear. One might almost say that the book is written so that anyone who might be interested in its application to his own particular concerns can hope to find something that bears on his needs.

PART 1

Mutation and the Concept of Intrinsic Mutagenesis

CHAPTER 1

THE TWO IMPERATIVES

The two basic evolutionary needs of all species of higher animal are survival to reproductive age, and death when survival offers no reproductive advantages to the species. The thesis of this essay is that both requirements are solved genetically by methods which involve control of mutability in the broad sense. For survival there must be an adequate appearance of mutants to ensure possibilities of adjusting to changes in the ecosystem or occupying any new ecological niches which may become available. It is, however, just as important biologically that the old generation should be discarded as soon as the new one is established. The mechanism is that of senescence, by which, once reproductive performance is completed, ageing develops almost certainly by the progressive acceleration of somatic mutation. Either by way of increasing vulnerability to environmental impacts or by intrinsically developed disease (cancer, etc.), death eventually ensues.

There is no escape from the conclusion that survival and continuing evolution on the one hand and an average lifespan for the individual appropriate to the species on the other are dependent on the occurrence of mutation. It is axiomatic to modern biology that mutation is a wholly random process in so far as the nature of the resulting change in genetic 'information' is concerned. Any *control* of mutation can only be in the form of modification in one direction or the other of the rate of mutation. It becomes inescapable, then, for us to postulate that the rate of germ-line mutation in the species and of somatic mutation in the individual must have optimal values for each particular species. If those two statements are, as I suggest, axiomatic, the two sets of mutation rates must be determined genetically; their regulation is just one of the responsibilities laid on the nucleotide sequences of the genome. My central thesis is that lifespan is one of the genetically determined aspects of every vertebrate organism and that it is mediated by genetic control of the rate of somatic mutation throughout the cells of the body most importantly perhaps in those cell lines that are subject to continued clonal proliferation throughout life. Basically I want to examine the justification for a concept of *intrinsic mutagenesis*, a means by which the species, and in a sense the individual, can control the rate of mutation in both germ-line and somatic nuclei to its evolutionary advantage.

For reasons which most biologists are willing to accept, there is a broad identity of the processes of mutation in viruses, in bacteria, in sexually reproducing metazoa and in parthenogenetic ones. At the mammalian level, which is our almost exclusive interest, this holds for both germ-line cells and somatic cells. There are infinite differences in detail, in the form in which results of mutation are expressed, and how they can be experimentally demonstrated, but a single statement will cover all types of mutation: it is a change in the molecular structure of a segment of DNA which (*a*) is compatible with continued replication of the segment and the viability of the organism or cell affected, and (*b*) is transmitted to all descendant genomes according to the rules of genetics appropriate to the organisms concerned.* Primary discussion of mutation can be based on that general definition, always provided that we add the qualification that in all natural circumstances mutation is rare and, as far as information in the genome is concerned, at random. Rare, random, and indefinitely transmissible structural alterations in DNA—almost every word in that phrase needs some expansion before we can approach the real problems of ageing and its associated diseases. Perhaps the random character of mutation provides the best starting point.

The random element in biology

For over a hundred years the implications of Darwinian evolution have been progressively elucidated and over the period there has been an

* In viruses without DNA, mutation can occur in the RNA, which for them is the sole primary repository of genetic information. Errors of the same quality occur in the RNA of bacterial and mammalian cells, but on the classical view such changes can never be transmitted to descendant cells and cannot therefore give rise to mutations. With the discovery of reverse transcriptases by which information carried on RNA can be used to guide DNA synthesis, the possibility of exceptions to that rule must remain open

increasing grasp of the intensely random character of the processes concerned. We come into very difficult country when we speak about random regularities. It is a field about which I have no philosophical or mathematical competence to speak, but only a biologist's superficial familiarity with the concept. What concerns me is the experience that, what looked at individually are wholly random occurrences, when collected in large enough numbers generate reproducible regularities which are subject to mathematical formulation and scientific analysis.

One can speak of an individual gas molecule colliding with another at some specific angle of contact and thereon changing in course and velocity in a fashion as deterministic in principle as a collision between two billiard balls. In every practical and experimental consideration, however, the individual trajectories and collisions of the molecules are all subsumed into temperature, pressure and volume, which can undergo interrelated changes in the simple deterministic fashion of elementary physics. In genetics, the situations are much more complex, but there are many occasions in genetics where the result that emerges to determine the quality of a new individual can be legitimately compared to the fall of a hand from a well shuffled pack of cards, or the sequence of black and white balls drawn blindfold from a barrel.

It would be impossible and inappropriate to attempt an elementary outline of genetics here, but one example indicating random disposition of genetic information can be given. If we take A, B, C, etc. to represent units of specific genetic information (genes) in a certain chromosome, we know that they are linearly arranged in some form of thread-like structure

A B C D E F G H I J . . .

and that each unit or group of units is responsible for determining the quality of some component of the structure or functional activity of the organism. The sequence of genes, in other words, carries the information that will be expressed in a range of bodily qualities (phenotypic characters); any change in the nature of the genes will be reflected in a corresponding phenotypic change in the organism. In the process by which one of two sets of information passes from each parent to offspring there is an important function referred to as crossing over, which can be represented schematically, as in Figure 1.

Without going into detail, the whole study of crossing over and the identification of the actual linear order of genetic units depends on accepting the axion that the switch point shown in the example between

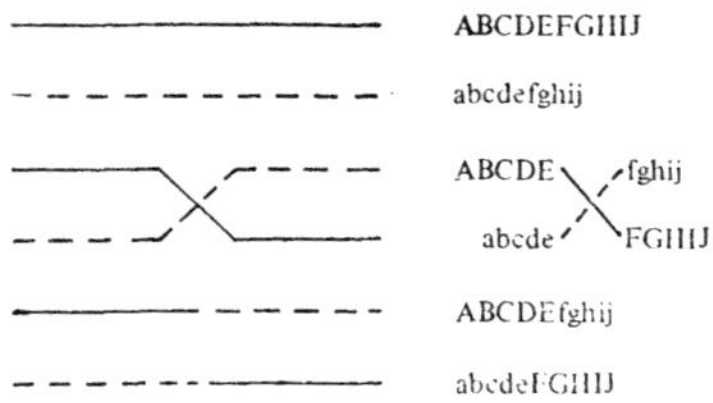

Figure 1 Crossing over. When two chromosomes break and change partners, the position of the break—here between E and F—is wholly random

E and F is equally likely to occur at any other point in the sequences. As far as the geneticist is concerned, the decision is a wholly random one.

Genetics is concerned with (*a*) the precise reproduction of parental characters in the offspring, (*b*) the random reassortment of qualities in which the parents differ, and (*c*) the appearance of new genetic information, which can just as validly be described as the intrusion of error into (*a*). In the first process we are dealing with certainty. When a non-sexual organism like a bacterium multiples, 999 out of 1000 descendants are accurate copies in all essential respects of the ancestral form. The sexual process which alone introduces (*b*) (recombination and crossing over) involves reassortment without change in the units. The random aspect concerns only the reassortment. Introduction of novelty or of error can best be exemplified in the simple asexual multiplication of a bacterium. Here it is expedient to work not with the gene itself but with the subunits, the nucleotide pairs, that in linear array make up the DNA of the genes. The commonest form of mutation, the so called point mutation, involves a change in one of these nucleotide subunits of a gene. If we take not a series of genes but a set of subunits making up a gene and again label them in linear order, A B C D E F G H I J . . . , 999/1000 will reproduce precisely the same sequence, but in the 0.1 per cent we would find an immense variety of random errors, each of which could in principle be identified experimentally. We might find, for instance, a relatively common change—1 in a million perhaps—where D was changed to Δ, and as a result the *mutant* bacterium required an extra vitamin before it could grow. The number of mutations, of errors and changes in the information, that can be obtained from the descendants of a single bacterium of that very common type, *Escherichia coli*, is probably unlimited. Many thousands of mutant form of *E. coli* have been isolated and the position of the change in the information sequence established. There are elaborate maps of the endless circular strand of DNA that is the equivalent of a chromosome in *E. coli* in which every point on the circumference has its label. There is no limit to the work that can be done, and every year or two the maps have to be made with larger circles to carry more and more labels.

Each labelled unit has its own chemical character and each is reproduced accurately in the vast majority of instances, but in one way or another each is subject to accident and error. For the most part, error strikes at random; any unit is as likely to be involved as any other, even when the overall incidence of error is increased, for example, by irradiating the culture with X-rays or ultraviolet light. This is not to say that the chemical action is at random. Irradiation with ultraviolet light, for example, produces a special type of damage described as thymine-dimerization, and most mutations it produces seem to arise as a result of error in the process of repairing the primary damage. The chemical and enzymatic processes are well defined, but a damaged pair of adjacent thymines can be present in any segment of DNA, in any gene of the whole genome. It may be chemically determinate, but informationally it is at random.

When the dynamics of mutation are studied in *E. coli*, quite accurate estimates of the frequency of any mutation which is experimentally convenient to handle can be made. The rate of mutation is always small and will usually lie between 10^{-5} and 10^{-9}. As a very rough estimate, one may take Szilard's figure that the average likelihood that one of the bases in DNA will be changed by 'point mutation' is around 10^{-8} for each replication of the genome. This will give at least an approximate idea of the rarity of mutation.

Has mutation a cause?

Once a phenomenon is recognized, it is natural to seek a cause. No one seriously doubts that only the regular or irregular occurrence of mutations has made evolution possible. Those who are interested in the origin of cancer speak with many voices, but hardly any would dispute that on the basis of the definition I have given of mutation all cancers result from somatic mutation. Necessarily there has been much discussion of the cause of mutation.

Most discussion takes as its starting point the established fact that certain physical and chemical agents can greatly increase the rate of mutation in some experimental test object—most often *E. coli*, but sometimes the fruit-fly, *Drosophila*, or the laboratory mouse. Within the last decade increasing use has been made of mammalian cell cultures, often of human origin. With an appropriate dose of ionizing radiation or of certain mutagenic chemicals any of these test objects will show a heightened mutation rate. It is well known that to double the spontaneous rate of mutation one must use a relatively large dose of radiation—around a thousand times as much as would be received from a normal environment in a year. Mutagenic chemicals that have more than a trivial effect may belong to many different structural types. No one seems to have been able to find any chemical quality that is common to all mutagens. Many of them are also capable of producing cancer in laboratory animals, and particularly for those like myself, who believe that the basis of cancer is somatic mutation, it is common to think of mutagens and carcinogens as a single category of agents, differing only in the way by which their activity is studied in the laboratory. Most such agents are synthetic substances which have never formed a significant component of the biosphere, but there are a few, such as caffeine and aflatoxin, which are produced by plants or fungi. Probably most biochemists and geneticists would consider that any type of molecule or ion that can react with DNA or with the various enzymes connected with its duplication or other functions is a potential mutagen. For obvious evolutionary reasons such substances are either very rare in nature or are effectively prevented from reaching the active DNA of an organism. The few chemical mutagens or carcinogens known to exist in any natural environment are in concentrations of only a few parts per billion. For them also the 'doubling dose', no matter how small it may appear in milligrams, is many thousands of times larger than any possible natural concentration.

The early tendency to look for a cause of mutations in cosmic rays and the other components of background radiation from radioactive elements in the environment is by no means wholly extinct, but there is no conceivable way by which 'background' can be responsible for more than a very small proportion of the spontaneous mutations that are observed. Equally, there is no evidence of the existence of chemical mutagens in anything approaching an adequate concentration in natural living environments. The most usual present day interpretation is that mutation is simply a result of random happenings at the level of thermal molecular movement. This is essentially a confession of ignorance, and from the nature of the hypothesis it is insusceptible to experimental test. If there is an alternative approach which is in principle subject to experimental disproof or verification, it should be formulated and tested.

On the hopeful assumption that the concept of intrinsic mutagenesis may interest some immunologists and gerontologists who are not deeply concerned with molecular genetics, it seemed appropriate to devote the next two chapters to an elementary account of fairly recent thought on the processes of DNA duplication and mutation. For obvious reasons, most of the material in both chapters is drawn from bacterial genetics.

CHAPTER 2

INTRINSIC MUTAGENESIS: AN ELEMENTARY DISCUSSION AT THE LEVEL OF MOLECULAR BIOLOGY

The DNA of any organism is incredibly complex, dynamic, and controlled. Segments of the double helix are continually being unwound and transcribed to RNA. Damage by radiation, by free radicals, and by chemical molecules reactive with DNA is constantly occurring. At intervals the whole fantastic process of mitosis, with all its possibilities of breaks, wrong connections, and so on, is initiated and completed. Every one of these functions requires the constant activity of enzymes, each functioning at the right place and the right time. How many enzymes there are, how they function, and how their amount, rate of synthesis, and specific localization are controlled—these are known in rather elementary outline for *E. coli*, with confirmation from some other bacteria. When specifically looked for, most of the enzymes defined for *E. coli* have been shown to be present in mammalian, including human, cells.

The key enzymes

The enzymes concerned include the following types, which have been defined almost wholly at the functional level, although several of the *E. coli* forms have been isolated as approximately pure molecular populations. Some of the proteins concerned seem to have more than one type of enzymatic activity and, conversely, two distinguishable proteins may appear to have the same, or a closely related, enzymatic function.

Monitoring enzymes
The process of repair, notably by the specific type of lesion (thymine dimerization) produced by ultraviolet light, must require some form of constant movement of an enzyme (an endonuclease) over each polynucleotide strand in order for it to 'know' where the lesion is and initiate the repair process. Then there are the restriction enzymes which can destroy any foreign DNA that may intrude into the genome. Here the process is interesting enough to justify a little detail in its description[1].

A restriction enzyme is only called into action when it recognizes a certain nucleotide sequence, usually a symmetrical one, that might be, for instance . . . X A C A X A C A X X . . . where X can be any type of standard nucletotide. Such a sequence must of course be 'forbidden' in the organism that produces the restriction enzyme in question It is a revealing instance of the random quality of biological pattern that any substantial segment of DNA will have every possible 5 or 6 unit sequence of the 4 nucleotides except those that are specifically forbidden. Any foreign DNA can therefore be recognized, but only if restriction enzymes are constantly patrolling every functionally active length of DNA in the genome. Everything underlines the importance of maintaining the integrity of every significant pattern of nucleotide sequence.

Endonucleases
These are enzymes which, as it were, make a cut at some desired spot in an intact segment of DNA, for example on either side of a dimer lesion produced by ultraviolet irradiation. Once the cut has been made, there are two free ends which thus become accessible to *exonucleases*, which, starting at one end (5′—OH) of any accessible chain, can progressively remove each successive unit as it becomes the end member of the chain. The liberated nucleotides presumably pass directly or indirectly into the metabolic pool of 'building stones', from which new sequences of DNA are built up by the next set of enzymes to be considered.

DNA polymerases
DNA polymerase (DP) is an enzyme or system of enzymes which is responsible for using a single strand of DNA as a template on which to construct a segment of a complementary strand, each nucleotide being added to the 3—C end of the growing strand in such a fashion

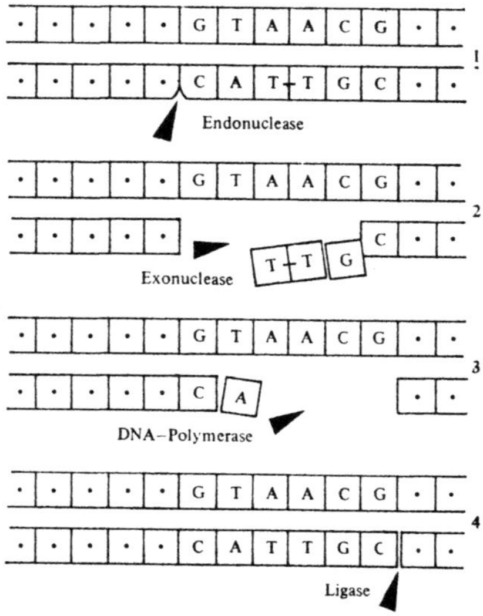

Figure 2 The process of DNA repair after damage by ultraviolet radiation.

1. The lesion, a thymine dimer, is recognized by an endonuclease and a primary incision made a few units away from the lesion.
2. An exonuclease then removes the segment containing the damage.
3. A DNA polymerase refills the gap with nucleotide units appropriate to the intact strand.
4. The repair is completed by the action of a DNA ligase

as to reconstitute the double-stranded structure of DNA. This may be part of the process of DNA duplication in the first phase of mitosis or one of the steps in DNA repair. In *E. coli* there are at least four differentiable DPs whose precise functions are still almost unknown. Study of mutants which over a particular range of temperature (*ts* mutants) do not allow replication of DNA has shown that at least six or seven loci can be involved. The product of one locus, *dna* E, has been identified as DPIII, which so far is the only enzyme known to be absolutely necessary for duplication of DNA and bacterial division to occur. The others may be basically indicative of the complex requirements needed to ensure the necessary degree of accuracy in getting the sequence right, whether in DNA duplication at mitosis or in repairing physiological breaks, or those resulting from micro-impacts from the environment. In view of the infinitely greater complexity, spatial and temporal, of mammalian somatic cells, one can be certain that the organization of genetic material is more complex and more intricately controlled than in any bacterial cell. For a variety of direct and indirect reasons one must picture a wide range of specifications for DPs in every somatic cell genome plus the appropriate machinery to call those required into action at the proper stage of differentiation or repair of the cell.

Ligases

The final step in any activity involving construction or reconstruction of a DNA segment to pattern is the action of an enzyme, a ligase, in finally linking the 3′—OH end of a newly organised segment to the appropriate stabilizing nucleotide.

The nature of mutation

A mutation results when an error occurs in the duplication or repair of a DNA component of such a nature that a persisting altered state develops which does not interfere with the capacity of the cell concerned to replicate and is transmitted regularly to all descendants of the mutant cell, subject to the ordinary rules of Mendelian genetics. The appearance of some observable altered quality in cell or organism (phenotypic expression of the mutation) will depend on the nature of the mutation and the factors discussed as dominance, penetrance and modification in classical genetics.

What must be emphasized is that a mutation is not a random chemical interference with DNA but the end result of a process leading to the reconstruction of a fully functioning genome. The relevant DNA segment may have an A–T nucleotide pair replacing the original G–C or a section of nucleotides may be deleted or reversed, but, except for the alteration in sequence pattern, the segment remains a perfectly normal piece of gentic mechanism, not a chemically traumatized one.

The basic facts about mutation in relation to what are referred to as standard physical and chemical mutagens are as follows:

1. All organisms, whether simple prokaryotes like bacteria or the most highly developed eukaryotes, with man as example, show a measurable rate of 'spontaneous' mutation which is much higher than could be accounted for by known 'mutagens' in the environment.

2. Application of high intensities of agents capable of inducing chemical change in DNA increases the number of mutations above the

spontaneous rate. The intensity necessary to double the rate can be judged from the approximate value of 200 R for X-irradiation, taken with the physical definition of 1 R as producing 1.6×10^{12} ion pairs, i.e. potentially damaging episodes, per gram.

3. Over a short range of intensities, from the lowest level where results can be clearly distinguished from the spontaneous level, upwards to the point of gross destructive action, there is an approximate linear relationship between dose and biological effect. It is impossible to determine experimentally whether this holds for doses significantly below those theoretically capable of producing an effect less than equivalent to the spontaneous rate.

4. With reagents specifically chosen for their reactivity with DNA, such as alkylating agents and acridines, a fairly precise account can be given of what probably happens in the (always small) proportion of bacteria or other cells that mutate. The two final changes, both requiring 'normalization' of the initial chemical effect by one or two sets of replication, are (*a*) replacement of one base pair by a different pair or (*b*) a 'frame-shift' resulting from the simple addition or deletion of a pair, a type of error usually occurring within a repetitive sequence of bases.

Possible interpretations of these facts are as follows:

I. Mutations result always from random damage by agents, known and unknown, capable of chemical interaction with DNA. A proportion of the damaging episodes result in inability of the DNA to replicate, which is necessarily equivalent to a lethal effect; another set undergoes repair and the segments are returned to normal. Neither of these results will be experimentally recognizable. Only intermediate types of damage can give rise to a persisting structural modification that becomes recognizable as a mutation.

II. Repair is so effective that most damage by mutagenic environmental agents is rapidly and effectively dealt with so far as repair to a viable form is possible. Any impact from a 'normal' environment is fully within the capacity for repair. Only grossly intense unbiological exposures produce results (mutations) because of inability of repair processes to give a satisfactory reproduction of former pattern in a proportion of the episodes of damage. The rate (or number) of mutations will remain linearly related to the intensity and duration of the damaging agent.

Alternatives I and II probably cover the interpretations of mutagenesis currently acceptable to the majority of geneticists. There is, however, a third possibility.

III. As will be discussed in the body of the book, there are fundamental biological requirements that a certain low but determinate level of mutation should be maintained (*a*) in the germ cell line to provide an optimal entry of novel information to allow the evolutionary plasticity needed for survival in an always changing ecosystem; and (*b*) in some or all somatic cell lines to allow a definable lifespan appropriate to the species. In the absence of sufficient information about most other organisms, this concept is for the time being applied only to man and other mammals.

The hypothesis will be elaborated that a determinate level of mutation rate, but not any qualitative determination of the type of mutation, could be established genetically by modification of the enzymes concerned to give an appropriate range of error propensity, allowing the fidelity with which DNA is duplicated to be set at the required level. For convenience, one could refer to the ratio between the number of nucleotide pairs accurately set to the number of wrong pairs as a measure of fidelity, with values perhaps from 10^{10} for highest fidelity to 10^4 for the lowest. This is a guess, based on Orgel's figure of 10^7 as the average value, and it should be self-evident that other enzymes than DNA polymerases could be concerned in determining overall fidelity. On such a view, the level of mutation will depend on the total number of enzymatic actions carried out by the DNA polymerase or other relevant enzymes. If DP action during repair of X-ray damage is very much greater than is involved in mitosis and both types of work are done with the same fidelity, there will naturally be a demonstrable increase in the number of mutant qualities expressed after irradiation.

* * *

The whole of the book is concerned with trying to decide between the currently orthodox interpretations I and II and the combination of II and III which offers the new approach that is being presented. Here it need only be said, first, that we have no measure of the mutation rate optimal for evolution, or at least that I am not sufficiently conversant with the literature on molecular evolution to be aware of possible rates. For somatic cells we have a potential measure by hypothesis in the lifespan of the species, which is regarded as a function of the fidelity of some or all of the key enzymes concerned in DNA duplication. On this basis the incidence of mutation would be accelerated in short-lived animals as compared with longer-lived species. Further experiment is needed, but the association of malignant disease, not with time but with senescence, already points strongly in that direction.

CHAPTER 3

MUTATOR GENES AND OTHER LEADS FROM BACTERIAL GENETICS

Ageing is not an aspect of bacterial existence, but the whole place in nature of bacteria depends on their capacity for mutation in many directions. Almost any change in the constitution of a nutrient medium in which a pure culture of bacteria is growing will very soon result in the appearance of a mutant population better suited to the new conditions. Even under optimal conditions of culture, mutation is constantly occurring, and for certain types of mutant there are highly convenient methods of measuring mutation rates.

Those rates can be increased by physical and chemical agents, and in the last two decades there has been a concentration of effort on interpreting the effect of such mutagens on the chemical structure of DNA. One favoured approach has been the use of base analogues, such as 5-bromuracil, which can replace a certain proportion of thymines. In such experiments a direct influence of the mutagen on the DNA can be demonstrated and a reasonable explanation of the mutations which can be detected after replication offered.

In bacterial and virus genetics, nitrous acid can also act as a powerful mutagen by its capacity to react with the bases themselves, converting adenine to hypoxanthine, guanidine to xanthine, and cytosine to uracil. Either directly or as a result of replication repair these can result in base-pair replacements.

In such cases where specific base changes are involved it is legitimate to accept the errors as being primarily dependent on the action of the mutagen rather than as errors arising with programmed frequency in the subsequent repair and replication processes.

Our concern, however, is with mutations produced spontaneously or by less specific physical and chemical mutagens. These may show a number of features which could be relevant to what occurs in somatic mammalian cells. Those to be discussed are specially relevant to the possible role that DNA polymerases may play in mutation.

The influence of manganous salts as mutagen

For rather personal reasons one of the findings that has most impressed me in this field was made in 1950 by Demerec[(2)], whom I knew well at Cold Spring Harbor. There were circumstances of interest, too, about how the significance of the experiments were recognized.

In an informal discussion with Professor Bruce Holloway at Monash University on mutation, he mentioned that for his work with *Pseudomonas aeruginosa* the use of manganous salts (following Demerec) had proved invaluable. For this organism, ultraviolet radiation had given a very poor yield of mutants, but dilute $MnCl_2$ was an excellent mutagen. This called to mind a recent abstract I had read of a paper by Springgate *et al.*[(3)], in which in the course of work on the significance of the Zn^{++} ion, which is an integral part of DNA polymerase of *E. coli*, they tested the ability of other divalent metal ions to replace the zinc. The apoenzyme had less than 5 per cent of the original activity which could be restored completely by Zn^{++}; it could regain 90 per cent by treatment with Co^{++} and 60 per cent with Mn^{++}. There was obviously a possibility that the manganous ion was mutagenic in virtue of its potential capacity to replace the physiological Zn ion in the metalloenzyme.

A detailed reading of Demerec and Hanson's 1951 paper provided us with a set of experiments which might have been deliberately designed to answer the question we were asking. A streptomycin-dependent strain (*E. coli* (B/r.SD4)) was tested for its capacity to produce non-dependent mutants after treatment with mutagenic chemicals. It was found that to obtain consistent positive results it was necessary to wash the bacteria with 0.15 M NaCl before exposing them to the standard 0.04 per cent $MnCl_2$ solution. Using this technique, the spontaneous mutation rate was extremely low ($1.4/10^8$), but with the $MnCl_2$ it rose to $5000–7000/10^8$. If the bacteria were washed in distilled water, only a few hundred mutants were obtained. In an attempt to analyse the significance of this difference, various other salts were used for the preliminary washing.

Table 1 is a summary of the relevant parts of the experiment in which 0.15 M solutions of chlorides of the metals shown were used to wash the bacteria before they were tested with the standard $MnCl_2$ solution as mutagen.

Table 1 Manganous salts as mutagen for *E. coli*

The table shows the effect of preliminary washing of the bacteria with the chlorides indicated (0.15 M) followed by exposure to 0.04 per cent $MnCl_2$ solution. (Data from Demerec and Hanson(2), by courtesy of *Cold Spr. Harb. Symp. quart. Biol.*)

Metal	*% survivors*	*Mutants/10*^{8}
Na	59	7108
K	50	6760
Ca	81	2890
Mg	91	18
Co	73	63
Zn	47	6

Preliminary washing with $ZnCl_2$ almost completely eliminated the powerful mutagenic effect of manganous ions. The findings are wholly compatible with the assumption that Mn^{++} acts by replacing Zn in a metalloprotein, presumably DNA polymerase. The preliminary washing with a much higher concentration of Zn^{++} ensured that the balance as between Zn and Mn was strongly in favour of the former and very little substitution of Zn in the enzyme occurred. Clearly that interpretation must be verified by the application of modern methods, and fuller information obtained about the metal content of any other enzymes involved. It is known for instance that DNA-dependent RNA polymerase of *E. coli* is also a Zn-containing enzyme(4).

In general terms, however, it can be said that a Zn-containing enzyme concerned with DNA replication becomes very error-prone when the Zn is replaced by Mn. Omitting any qualifications about lag in expressing the mutant character, about 1:20 000 show error in replication. Unlike most potent mutagens, there is only a trivial mortality as a result of its action, and limited tests showed that it was also an active mutagen in all the seven other experimental situations used. It therefore becomes a working hypothesis, which should be almost immediately available for test, that relatively minor changes in the three-dimensional configuration of an enzyme, by changing Zn to Mn, are sufficient to modify strikingly the fidelity of DNA replication.

It this is true, it greatly strengthens the broader hypothesis that point mutation in the gene coding for a DNA polymerase could also result in changes in the fidelity of action of the enzyme and on occasion raise the mutation rate to a level which would justify the gene being classed as a mutator gene.

Mutator genes in bacteria and bacterial viruses

Mutator genes are well known in *E. coli*, but a more illuminating example is found in regard to phage T4, one of the classical viruses pathogenic for *E. coli*. Speyer *et al.*[5] worked with a series of temperature-sensitive (*ts*) mutants of T4D, involving gene-43, known to code for a DNA polymerase specific for T4 and T6 but not effective with T3 or T5. Among these mutants some, but not all, increased the rate at which *r* mutants were produced. Standard stocks of T4 produce from 0.01–0.1 per cent of R mutants; one *ts* mutant, L56, gave nearly 50 per cent of mottled plaques which contained between 10 and 50 per cent of *r* mutants. Similarly, it produced approximately 100 times as many acridine-resistant or host range mutants. The mutator gene was shown to be at the gene-43 position in the genome, and revertants to temperature resistance had simultaneously lost their mutagenic capacity.

Drake and Allen[6] subsequently found, in working with similar material, two *anti-mutator* strains which strongly inhibited certain types of reversion induced by base analogues.

These experiments show that the proportion of error in DNA replication can be modified as a result of (point) mutations in the DNA polymerase of the phage. Bacterial viruses are genetically more labile than bacteria, but no one has suggested that their genetic mechanisms are fundamentally different from those of the organisms they parasitize. The whole process of their infection and multiplication in the bacterium demands such homology. If bacteriophage DNA polymerase can mutate to forms more and less prone to error than the wild type, we have the best possible justification for seeking, and expecting, the same capacity in all other DNA polymerases and any other equally *responsible* enzymes.

The details of the enzymes concerned with DNA replication and repair in *E. coli* still seem obscure to one who is not a member of the 'invisible college' concerned. The status of Kornberg's enzyme, DNA polymerase I, suffered a blow when De Lucia and Cairns[7] obtained a mutant lacking the enzyme. In a recent summary, Cairns[8] points out that, until fairly recently, crudities of technique ensured that all the DNA polymerase reactions being studied were repair actions and DNA polymerase I is now known to be primarily, and perhaps exclusively, a repair enzyme. Two other polymerases, II and III, have been characterized on physical and enzymological grounds. Since mutants lacking II can exist, III is presumed to be the essential DNA replicase. This has been confirmed by the isolation of a mutant with a thermosensitive, DNA polymerase III. Such mutants fail to replicate DNA at the restrictive temperature[9].

Cairns sounds a warning that DNA synthesis is known to be a highly complex process, not proceeding continuously, but with numerous initiation points responsible for beginning separate 'Okazaki pieces', which are subsequently fused by a ligase. There is evidence that the starting point of each piece is a short section of newly synthesized RNA and a DNA-dependent RNA polymerase may be one of the components of the enzyme system responsible for DNA replication. In all probability further complexities await demonstration.

Several mutator genes have been described for *E. coli*, and what evidence is available strongly suggests that they act by modifying one or other DNA polymerase. The first was obtained by Treffers' group[10] in 1954 (*mut T1*) and has been extensively worked with since. Yanowsky *et al.*[11], studying the structure of mutant forms of tryptophan synthetase, Protein A, concluded that the action of the mutator gene was by transversion of A–T to G–C and was unidirectional. This points to a modified DNA polymerase. They point out, however, that there are other possibilities, notably the production of base analogues distorting DNA function. Siegel and Bryson[12] note that mutator genes are not necessarily all at the same locus and that a new one, *mut S1*, increased the frequency of phage resistance, which *mut T1* did not. Hill[13] showed a synergistic effect of an *E. coli* mutator gene (*mut H1*) on mutagenesis by ultraviolet radiation and alkylating agents. It was at a different map locus from the conventional DNA polymerase region, but could be associated with a different polymerase.

The synergistic effect offers a strong suggestion that both ultra-violet and chemical mutations are induced indirectly and depend essentially on the relative efficiency of the DNA repair enzymes and the fidelity with which the original correct situation is restored.

Repair of bacterial DNA

In describing the process of dark repair of ultraviolet damage to DNA in *E. coli*, Gunther Stent[(14)] contends that one or more enzyme molecules must be constantly moving round the entire circle of the bacterial genome to monitor the double-stranded DNA for anomalies such as the pyrimidine dimers resulting from ultraviolet radiation. When a lesion is recognized, this nuclease makes two cuts, a few nucleotides on either side, and another nuclease removes the intervening portion of the strand involved. The gap is filled by a DNA polymerase, using the uninvolved strand as template, and a ligase joining the two ends completes the process. Exposure of DNA to X-rays *in vivo* or *in vitro* causes breaks which in general are mended within minutes, sometimes by a simple ligase action, but with excision of segments with damaged bases if necessary. Repair mechanisms, often of considerable complexity, have been demonstrated for most of the chemical agents capable of damaging DNA. Howard-Flanders[(15)] refers to investigations on the excision of products of alkylation reactions and subsequent repair. Where both strands of DNA are damaged, often with fusion, an elaborate post-replication repair, involving the use of a duplex strand as template, is described. The 'objective' is always the faithful reconstruction of the pattern as it was before damage, and everything suggests that the potentialities for accurate repair will be extended rather than diminished by future research.

In view of our central theme of intrinsic mutagenesis being characteristic of both normal DNA replication and of DNA repair processes, it is interesting to quote Howard-Flanders on ultraviolet-mutations in bacteria. 'It has been suggested that occasional errors in gap-filling might be responsible for the mutagenic effects of ultraviolet light and that post replication repair is an error-prone system. This theory is supported by two observations: (i) ultraviolet mutagenesis appears to follow DNA replication and (ii) it requires both rec A^{+} and lex A^{+} genes which control replication and repair.'

The lessons from bacterial genetics

The leading impression to a non-specialist from a foray into the recent literature on those aspects of bacterial genetics which seemed to be relevant is of the subtlety, complexity and fidelity of the processes concerned. The existence of restriction enzymes is an example of the subtleties that can develop in the reactions that ensure the integrity and precise conformity to pattern of the genetic mechanisms. The coordination of endonuclease, exonuclease, DNA polymerase, and ligase in the recognition, excision and repair of a DNA lesion produced by the standard extrinsic mutagens is well established in bacteria, but at least to the uninitiated bespeaks an integrated complexity of interactions that exhausts the imagination. The fidelity of DNA replication is vouched for in the control mutation rate in any quantitative experiment with extrinsic mutagens. Less than 100 per 10^8 duplications is a usual figure, and even with a potent mutagen like ultraviolet radiation the yield is rarely increased by more than two orders of magnitude.

Another finding from bacterial genetics that is directly relevant to the broader theme is the regularity of the results when the error-proneness of the enzyme is increased, as in our instance where Zn is replaced with Mn. From the control average of $1.4/10^8$, optimal conditions with $MnCl_2$ gave values of $4–8000/10^8$. Random errors generated within any uniform system of adequate size must take on a stochastic regularity which can be expressed in a cellular population as mutation rate, but could in principle also be assessed from any observable result of those mutations such as lifespan or the age-specific incidence of cancer.

The importance of bacterial genetics for ageing theory must necessarily be very indirect. At most it can serve as a model for the human or mammalian situation in regard to those aspects of theory that are in terms of genetic concepts. It is not likely that much more can be gained from analysing the facts about human lifespan at a genetic level than a certainty that there is a significant genetic component; this is similarly evident in comparing mammalian species or the distinct strains of domesticated mammals. The subsequent development of an hypothesis as to the way the genetic requirement is mediated has to be initially an effort of the imagination—a working hypothesis that can help to sort out the available information and stimulate the planning of an experimental approach. Genetic experiments with mammals are only possible at a rather unsophisticated level. There is no conceivable way to test directly that the overall rate of somatic mutation in a mammalian species can be controlled by the structure of the key enzymes of DNA replication as determined by the corresponding germ-line genes. Whether or not such a mechanism exists may never be finally established. The most that can be hoped for is to strengthen the hypothesis progressively: (*a*) by establishing the existence of analogous processes in more easily handled biological models of which bacteria, viruses and other microorganisms are the most convenient; (*b*) to use cell cultures from the mammal being studied as a model one step closer to the primary object; and (*c*) to assess the usefulness of the hypothesis in throwing light on currently obscure aspects of relevant physiological or pathological phenomena in the primary object of study.

The three requirements will need to be pursued in parallel. Work on the model system of bacteria and viruses has already gone far beyond anything that could be envisaged in mammalian cells, but perhaps a gerontologist, more particularly a cytologist concerned with a gerontological problem, might well find new questions to ask his colleagues in bacterial genetics. If the suggestion cited earlier is correct, that replacement of Zn by Mn in the metalloenzyme greatly increases its mutator function as DNA polymerase, an important lead to the means by which error-proneness is adjusted might be developed. One gathers that simply from its intrinsic interest very intensive work is under way on the enzymes, ancillary proteins and modus operandi of DNA synthesis and repair in bacteria, and a rather precise statement of the processes may soon be available. This should be invaluable in guiding work in mammalian fields.

As indicated in the quotation from Howard-Flanders, there is already recognition by bacterial geneticists of the likelihood that the mutagenic action of physical and chemical agents does not depend on direct alteration of the DNA of the genome but is an indication of error in the repair function of the enzymes. In other words, the part played by the extrinsic mutagen may often be simply to increase the number of opportunities when errors can be made by the cells' own enzymes to a degree dependent on their inbuilt proneness to error.

CHAPTER 4

MUTATION IN EVOLUTION

The concept of intrinsic mutagenesis is no more than a formal expression for the opinion that the commonly accepted environmental causes of mutation are in normal circumstances quantitatively unimportant and for the most part effective only through their influence on the errors in DNA replication of intrinsic origin. Under these circumstances it is inevitable that discussion should centre first on the most readily measured mutagen and the one with the strongest emotional impact: ionizing radiation. The whole world is conscious of the danger associated with military and peaceful uses of atomic energy, and, like most senior biologists with some interest in public affairs, I have taken some part in official or semi-official discussion in this field. Always the controversy has centred on the question of the level of exposure that is safe, in the sense of producing no medically significant mutations or other genetic anomalies and no leukaemia or other form of neoplastic disease. In 1973 there was strong opposition to the expansion of the nuclear power industry in North America, and in Australia and the rest of the southern hemisphere equally fervent resentment at the atmospheric tests of nuclear devices in French territories in the Pacific. The problem is in principle highly relevant to the present theme and calls for a fairly detailed discussion.

The concept of a threshold

Every biologist dealing with very low levels of radiation that make only a fractional increase in the normal 100 milli-R* per annum of background radiation finds himself in the fundamental difficulty that there is no possible way yet discovered of determining objectively whether levels of radiation as low as those resulting from distant bomb tests have any biological effect at all. We know that very large doses of ten to a hundred times the total amount of radiation coming from our environmental background over a human lifetime can have damaging effects which can be measured. Statistically there is, as would be expected, a greater effect from a large dose than from a smaller one, and the convention has developed of assuming that a linear dose-effect relationship exists over the whole range of doses down to the smallest.

Perhaps the best example to offer concerns the effect of ionizing radiation in producing leukaemia. For a long period in England and elsewhere it was standard practice for the disease of the spinal column known as ankylosing spondylitis to be treated with large, repeated doses of therapeutic X-rays over the affected region. This necessarily involved irradiating a considerable fraction of the body. In time the radiologists began to recognize that a proportion of the patients who had been under treatment for several years developed leukaemia. It was still only a very small proportion, but many more than would be expected from the same number of untreated people of the same age. A long series of investigations was undertaken in England with a final report by Court Brown and Doll in 1965[16, 17]. This work involved more than 14 500 patients who had received large doses of X-rays approximately in the range 250 to 2500 R over the spinal column. In the group there were 52 cases of chronic myelogenous leukaemia or acute leukaemia instead of the 5.5 who would be expected in a control series. There was an approximate relationship between the amount of X-rays received and the likelihood of leukaemia, and the conclusion was reached that, in round figures, a total dose of 1000 R units was likely to give rise to about 5 cases per annum over ten or twelve years for each 10 000 men so treated.

To round off the figures and simplify what is really a very complex situation, we can say that a total dose of 1000 R produces leukaemia in 0.5 per cent of those who receive it. On the linear dose–effect rule a lifetime's exposure to one-tenth R per annum, say 5 R, would give a likelihood of one person in 40 000 developing leukaemia as a result. The

* The physical unit of ionizing radiation, the *roentgen*, needs to be modified for technica use in regard to biological effects, and two related units, *rad* and *rem*, are used. For my purpose the differences are immaterial and it is convenient to label the unit R, and the thousandth part of the amount a milli-R

process of calculating the quantitive effect of a small dose of ionizing radiation is both tedious and exasperating. It is always necessary to make quantitative assumptions for which only very slight factual justification is available and the end result will have to be expressed as a wide range of possibilties. This refers of course to calculations made on the basis of the linear dose–effect rule. To make things even more difficult, we know that almost every agent capable of producing biological damage has a threshold. Heat, electric shock, carbon monoxide, mercury salts can be thought of as examples. Below a certain intensity or a certain dose no harm is done. Although this is not yet officially accepted it seems likely that it holds also for all or most types of ionizing radiation. At least we can be certain that very low doses have less than a proportional effect, even if it is not quite zero.

In late 1972 two authoritative reports were issued, one by an international committee for the United Nations[18], and one, 'the BEIR report', by an official American committee[19]. Both discuss the problem of low doses of radiation in detail on the basis of experimental studies on a wide range of biological test objects. Both pay much attention to the evidence that there is an elaborate mechanism by which certain key enzymes monitor DNA for damage and repair it when necessary. Both reports reach the same conclusion that there is no decisive evidence for the existence of a threshold, that no direct evidence of harm by less than 25–30 R has ever been demonstrated, but that it is still a possibility that a linear dose–effect (LDE) relationship extends down to mimimal levels. All estimates of harm are therefore calculated on what we can call the LDE rule on the certainty that this is the 'worst possible' result. Unfortunately this has always resulted in the public assumption that this worst possible result is what in fact will happen.

Probably many workers in radiobiology would support an alternative approach, just as adequately backed by factual evidence, by which action was based on the statement on page 1 of the BEIR report. 'Exposure to man-made radiation below the level of background radiation will produce additional effects that are less in quantity and no different in kind from those which man has experienced and has been able to tolerate throughout his history.'

From our point of view the important information required is what proportion of the genetic anomalies or neoplastic conditions which occur in normal human populations could be ascribed to background radiation on the assumption that the LDE rule held over the whole range of doses. For the purposes, I have taken the lowest figure calculated on the LDE rule in the BEIR report for each type of known or suspected genetic disability. Table 4 on page 57 of the BEIR report, simplified in this fashion, is here shown as Table 2. The important finding is that if we

Table 2 Genetic damage in a population of one million

Disease or disability per million	*Current incidence*	*Effect of background, 5 R per generation*	
		First generation	*Equilibrium*
Dominant diseases	10 000	50	250
Chromosomal and recessive diseases	10 000	Slight	Slow increase
Disease and disability with partial genetic bases	40 000	5	50
Total	60 000	60(–1000)	300(–7500)

Data from the BEIR report[19], using the lowest value for the effect of background radiation (see text), except in giving the total effect where the calculated maximal effect is also shown (in brackets). By courtesy of U.S. Government Printing Office.

accept the lowest calculation as the most likely, the effect of continued exposure to an amount equal to background radiation is between 200 and 1000 times less than the *known* current incidence.

At this stage we are simply accepting without discussion that malignant disease, specifically leukaemia, is a manifestation of somatic mutation induced by iozining radiation in a small proportion of the cells of the bone marrow. A closer consideration of the relationship of somatic mutation to malignant change will be found in Chapters 12 and 13. However, it is appropriate to refer forward to Table 5 (see page 133) for a similar simplification of American findings on leukaemia and cancer in general. Here the caluculations indicate that 1–5 per cent of the cases of leukaemia could be due to radiation, but it is just as valid to emphasize that 95–99 per cent cannot be due to radiation.

Clearly the two relevant types of human disability, genetic anomaly and neoplastic disease, are both much too frequent to be ascribed to background radiation, the only universally present environmental agent that could reasonably be thought of as a *cause* of either condition. Much more discussion will be needed in relation to leukaemia and cancer, but for the present we can concentrate on the conclusion which seems to be generally accepted, that, as far as mutation functions as an evolutionary factor, it is almost wholly intrinsic to the organism. On the LDE rule, any effect, mutational or neoplastic, at around background levels will involve only a few individuals per million exposed. There is no conceivable way by which such effects can be recognized in human populations, nor is it a practical proposition to look for one additional death or mutation in a hundred thousand carefully tended and individually studied mice. There is no scientific basis for any conclusion on the effect of such levels of ionizing radiation; those published are simply a manifestation of what is politically and socially expedient in the temper of the times.

A more likely guess, but still one based on indirect evidence and analogy, is that, like every other environmentally damaging agent, the effect becomes minimal or zero as concentration falls below a certain threshold, and that this could probably lie somewhere between two and ten times the average background level. From our point of view such a

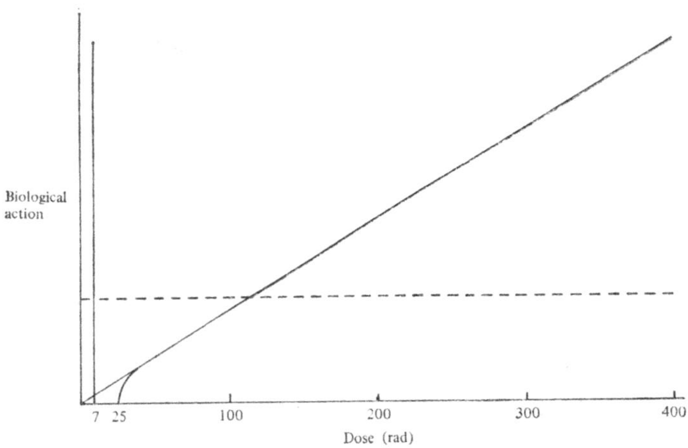

Figure 3 The LDE rule of the biological effect of radiation. Dose of radiation received is shown horizontally in rads. 7R is the total amount of 'background radiation' received in a lifetime, 25 R is the smallest amount that has ever been shown to have a demonstrable biological effect. Biological effect—either the production of mutations or the development of leukaemia or cancer—is shown vertically. The dotted line indicates the spontaneous occurrence of mutations or tumours in human populations. This is very much greater than anything that could conceivably be produced by exposure to background or several multiples thereof. The sloping line represents the linear dose–effect rule. The dark line is based on experimental observations, but what happens where the line is thin can never be directly observed. It may show a threshold with no action below about 25 R or it may show the LDE rule throughout.

This is a greatly simplified diagram, but it accurately indicates the nature of the problem.

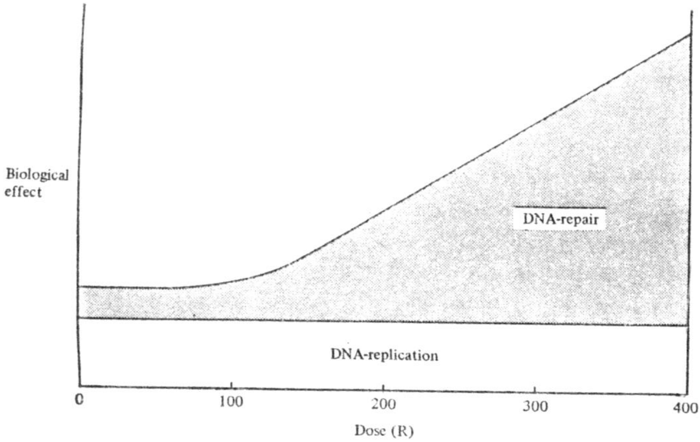

Figure 4 An alternative interpretation of the dose–effect relationship based on the concept of intrinsic mutagenesis. Here the observable line is as in Figure 3. The effect is, however, ascribed wholly to intrinsic error in replication or repair of DNA. The influence of mutagenic radiation is due to the greatly increased requirement for repair as the dose increases beyond 30 to 50 R. The part played by error in the repair processes is indicated by the shaded area

postulate would imply that in the course of evolution means have been developed to counter any damaging effect of the levels of ionizing radiation characteristic of the environment. Those levels have certainly varied over the three to four thousand million years of evolution and in the earliest stages much have been considerably higher than at present; the need for the evolution of effective mechanisms of DNA repair and the like would be correspondingly more urgent. An account has already been given of the extent and effectiveness of the repair mechanisms in *E. coli* and, by implication, their equal or greater effectiveness in mammalian cell. It may be many years before a firm, scientifically based statement can be made, but on present indications we cannot possibly ascribe the humanly harmful effects of somatic mutation to background levels of ionizing radiation. The hypothesis of their origin from some intrinsic mechanism remains open.

There are, however, potential chemical mutagens in the natural environment, and some thought must be given to the possibility that substances taken into the body in food, water or air may be responsible for the spontaneous mutations and cancers that we observe. It is known that minute amounts of some carcinogens are present in normal diets;

polycyclic hydrocarbons, aflatoxin, and nitrosamines are found in the order of a small number of parts per billion[20]. In addition, there are the vast number of organic chemicals of non-biological origin which are included as food additives for various purposes and an almost equally large number of substances used in industry which may be taken in unwittingly in air, water or food. All such possible mutagens (or carcinogens) have become steadily more numerous and all-pervasive since the beginning of this century. If they are dangerous, one should expect that an increasing incidence of dominant mutations and of cancer should have become evident between 1900 and 1970.

Abnormalities now recognized as genetic, such as various forms of dwarfism, have been known throughout history, and I know of no evidence that the incidence of genetic disease has increased in this century. Nor, with the conspicuous and well understood exception of primary lung cancer, is there any evidence that the incidence adjusted to age of the other forms of cancer has increased since 1900. Any carcinogenic (mutagenic) effect of material in food or drink would be expected to be reflected in gastric cancer or tumours of the liver. None is evident, and gastric carcinoma has been becoming considerably less common in Western countries, particularly in the United States of America.

There may still be an unexpected recognition of some environmental source of carcinogens-mutagens to account for the high spontaneous incidence of genetic anomalies and malignant disease. As the situation stands, however, there is a strong prima facie case for an intrinsic origin of the great majority of both types of anomaly. This is the first major postulate of the hypothesis of ageing that seems to be emerging from modern studies: that mutation in the restricted sense and the various manifestations of somatic mutation, including malignant disease, are not the effects of environmental agents impinging on the organism from outside, but arise within the organism.

It is a reasonable and widely accepted assumption that for any given type of evolving organism there will be an optimal rate for mutation and any other genetic processes which are responsible for the appearance of new phenotypes that can be tested for survival. During the three billion years of evolution there has been world enough and time to perfect any mechanism within the potentiality of living substance that has seemed to be needed for survival. The means has in principle always been the same. Error in the process of conservative replication has been constantly tested for novelty, and whenever novelty provided some advantage, however small, in selective survival, it has been seized upon and incorporated into the gene pool of the species whenever chance and circumstance would permit. I follow Monod[21] and his great precursors, Haldane, Fisher, Huxley, Dobzhansky and Mayr, in accepting no place in biology for anything beyond chance and necessity. In particular, there is no place for any end-directed process by which an organism can be improved according to a plan. In Monod's words, 'Destiny is written as and while, not before, it happens'. It may be too cumbersome never to speak in teleological terms, but whenever we do, the limitations of the evolutionary process must always be kept in mind. Those limitations may be specially hard to grasp when they concern the control of the very process itself. We are postulating a control of one random set of processes by another, equally random process.

Molecular interpretation

In attempting to devise an explanation of ways by which the frequency and extent of mutation might be modified—i.e. in providing an hypothesis at the molecular level for a function that is biologically required—I shall undoubtedly be influenced by my immunological background. In any living organism of the complexity of a warm-blooded vertebrate, effective moment to moment functioning requires much interchange of specific information. In the present context we can omit the workings of the central nervous system and concentrate on simpler systems by which circulating cells or soluble substances carry messages/instructions from one part of the body to another. A hormone from the pituitary 'instructs' the thyroid to increase its activity, or an anitgen from some site of infection calls for appropriate immunocytes to counter the infection. There are a thousand other types of analogous activity. In each, the specificity is controlled by mutual pattern recognition of large molecules.

On the messenger or effector molecule there is a certain atomic configuration, a steric pattern, that is complementary to the pattern of the specific receptor on the cell which is to be stimulated. The two molecular patterns, if properly oriented, will develop a non-covalent linkage dependent on the complementarity of their patterns. If that linkage has sufficient firmness (affinity), it will result in the generation of a signal that calls the needed cellular process into action.

In immunology particularly, this type of mutual recognition is often compared to a lock-key relationship. It is a useful simile, but it misses one very important point. There is no absolute specificity of the fit between two informational molecules. There can be minor differences on either side which will result in the mutual fit being 'good' or 'not so good' rather than a clear 'union' or 'no union'. To some extent the goodness of fit can be measured by the physical 'affinity' of the union, but additional qualitative factors may also be important. Whenever the effector or receptor substance is a protein, this soft-edged relationship holds. Any protein can undergo an infinity of changes, from minimal modification to a complete change in specificity by amino-acid residue replacements in the significant parts of the molecule. Such changes at the biological level can only result from mutational or equivalent changes in the controlling structural gene. A minor mutation with a minor modification in the pattern of the active group of any enzyme may, for instance, render the enzyme just a little less efficient than normal. When it is responsible for one phase of a finely coordinated activity, error in that activity may become more frequent. If the enzyme is concerned with the critical phases of DNA replication and the process of protein synthesis, inefficiency will be multiplied by secondary errors involving the structure of other enzymes.

To be a little more specific, we assume that all repairs to DNA, including physiological 'cut and mend' processes in the course of crossing over, are the responsibility of a series of closely coordinated enzymes and that any inefficiency will result in an increased number of mutations through failure of the repair to reconstitute normality. More broadly, the relative proportion of errors could, in principle, be modified in various ways by minor structural differences in the several enzymes concerned with cut and mend functions on DNA.

So far there is no evidence as to whether there is any control of mutability in the classical sense along these lines. We do not even know whether such a notoriously stable form as *Lingula*, which appears to have persisted unchanged for some hundreds of millions of years, is any less liable to mutation than a highly variable form like *Drosophila*. According to Dobzhansky[22], the average population of *Drosophila* in the wild has as large a burden of potentially harmful recessive genes as a human population. This could well be related to the need for genetic versatility to build up the variant populations that can occupy a wide variety of casual niches. On the other hand, the stability of *Lingula* may merely mean that it is so perfectly adapted to its standard environment that, no matter how mutable it may be, none of the mutations will be able to displace the standard form. It may take many years before geneticists can establish at a biological level the relative mutability of a range of animal forms, and considerably longer before they reach a molecular interpretation of the differences. The probability, however, is that such a control of mutability exists and that it has an evolutionary justification. If there are such genetic functions, mutability, from the random character of the errors giving rise to mutation, cannot be directed only in useful directions. Potentially valuable mutations can only arise amidst a vastly greater number of changes that are harmful in the sense that if they achieve expression the carriers of the mutant genes will be at a disadvantage for survival.

The association of mutator genes with DNA duplication in bacteria has already been described. It is known that mutants of *E. coli* and *B. subtilis* exist in which increased susceptibility to irradiation and/or higher mutability is associated with deficiency in DNA polymerase or other key enzymes concerned with replication and repair of DNA. This, on the one hand, suggests that modification of such enzymes could be a means of controlling mutation rate and, on the other, that the evolution of these repair enzymes may have been necessary to counter the effect of radiation from the environment. All experimental work on the biological effects of large doses of radiation suggests that the old axiom that damage is due to a single irreversible event in the cell is incorrect. Damage is always a multiple-hit process, readily modified by many factors, with everything to suggest a highly efficient machinery for dealing with chemical changes, single-strand breaks, and any other potentially harmful effects of a single ionizing event on DNA in the cell.

Under all the circumstances one feels justified in claiming that one of the chief problems that must have occupied evolution in the first two billion years of life's history was how to preserve the integrity of genetic information held as a single or double nucleotide strand that was always subject to the possibility of damage by ionization from penetrating radiation. In the last few years we have learnt a lot about the ways in which damage by ultraviolet radiation of bacteria can be repaired; the enzyme which recognizes and initiates deletion of the characteristic thymine-dimer lesion can only have arisen as a specific response to ultraviolet damage in early phases of the earth's history. Somewhat less is known about repair of DNA breaks induced by X-irradiation and other types of ionizing radiation, but the process is at least equally efficient and no doubt was evolved to neutralize an equivalent environmental hazard.

This discussion of mutation in evolution is only indirectly related to the theme of ageing; its function is to support the general thesis that somatic mutation is a basically similar process to both bacterial mutation and mutation at the germ-line level in higher organisms. The suggestion that modification of DNA polymerases or other key enzymes may be the process allowing intrinsic control of mutation rate can be elaborated more precisely in terms of somatic mutation.

CHAPTER 5

SOMATIC MUTATIONS

My own major interests in genetics were at first in relation to bacterial and animal viruses and more recently in various aspects of somatic mutation. Not altogether unreasonably, workers in the experimental biomedical sciences have resisted accepting hypotheses ascribing bodily phenomena, physiological or pathological, to somatic mutation. The objection was essentially that any hypothesis ascribing a phenomenon to a change taking place in a *single cell* is necessarily insusceptible to experimental test. By the time a demonstrable result, the production of a tumour or of a circulating antibody for instance, becomes available for investigation, there can be no direct evidence about the initiating process. This meant a corresponding freedom to ascribe the phenomenon to any type of somatic mutation that seemed to be expedient. To most experimental scientists any hypothesis which cannot in principle be proved wrong by appropriate experiment is regarded as irresponsible and illegitimate. What may well have been more important is the human tendency to prefer an explanation based on a specific cause and effect relationship rather than to accept a stochastic interpretation as adequate. This attitude is necessarily adopted by most experimental biologists, perhaps particularly by biochemists, and it is a historical fact that biomedical research in recent years has been dominated by people trained in biochemistry. The development of microbial chemistry as a branch of genetics in the 1940s led to molecular biology and an increasing interest by biochemists in genetic attitudes of thought. Even in the period 1958–1962, however, the concept of clonal selection(23), now generally accepted as the broad basis of immunological theory, was strongly resisted by most immunologists until the investigation of the monoclonal products of plasmacytomas (myeloma and Bence-Jones proteins) provided almost a categorical proof of its validity. The difficulty for most people was that there seemed to be a clear causal relationship between the immunizing infection or experimental injection and the appearance and specificity of the antibody response. It seemed evident to almost everyone that the antigen must somehow imprint a complementary quality on the immunoglobulin being synthesized in the cells concerned with antibody production. I had to struggle hard to remain convinced myself of the validity of the concept in view of the rather numerous experiments which were claimed to have disproved it between 1957 and 1965. Today the fact that the specific immune pattern, based on the variable segment of light and heavy chains, is genetically determined is taken as axiomatic. The controversies of the growing edge are now concerned with the nature of the genetic process by which diversity of pattern is generated in the somatic cell genome.

The cell culture approach

In recent years somatic mutation has become a more acceptable topic for laboratory study, thanks to the development of methods of demonstrating and measuring the frequency of mutation in mammalian cells in culture. Such cells have been freed from many of the constraints and controls of somatic cells in the mammalian body, but they are genuine somatic cells and, according to all the rules of biological experimentation, what is observed in cell cultures can be used with appropriate circumspection as a model for what happens or can happen to somatic cells *in vivo.*

Once methods of 'cloning' cells, i.e. of providing conditions by which a single cell would give rise to a colony of cells visible to the naked eye, had been developed by Puck and his successors[(24)], the techniques of the bacterial geneticists could be applied with only minor modifications. As in bacterial work, mutant cells which require some additional food factor to grow are common and of considerable biochemical interest. Such mutant cells can be isolated by making use of the fact that growing, but not quiescent, cells can be selectively poisoned by a toxic analogue of one of the DNA bases, bromodeoxyuridine (BUdR). The cells that have taken up the BUdR are killed by exposure to light, while those that failed to multiply because of some mutational deficiency remain alive. By appropriate use of enriched media, these can be made to grow and their particular deficiency analysed.

With this technique, and a variety of others when different types of mutation are sought, it can be shown that X-irradiation can produce mutation at a low but measurable rate. As an example, the mutation to a glycine-requiring mutant showed a rate per locus per R of 4×10^{-8}.

A simpler type of experiment is to determine the survival curve after exposure to various doses of radiation. The lethal effect of irradiation probably results from the same sort of physical damage as a detectable mutation and may be regarded as resulting from the induction of a lethal mutation owing to failure to repair the physical damage.

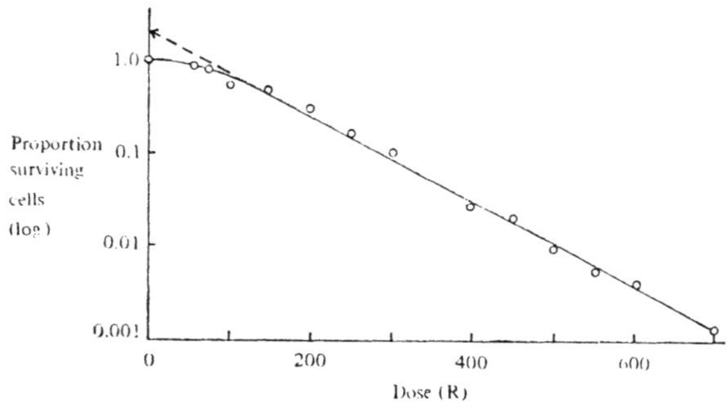

Figure 5 Irradiation of human cells in culture. The proportion surviving after graded doses is shown. Note the 'shoulder' showing that small doses have less than a proportional effect

Many such curves are available and all are of the same character (Figure 5), including experiments carried out on human lymphocyte cultures. When the percentage of surviving cells is plotted logarithmically against the dose, a straight line graph is obtained, apart from an initial 'shoulder', where there is less than proportionate action by the lowest doses. It has been shown that if a small dose, within the shoulder, is given and the cells allowed four hours incubation, they respond to a second set of irradiation as if the first episode had not occurred. If the interval is one hour or less, the effect of the two doses is additive. This is perhaps the clearest evidence of a repair process, and it is probably unimportant in principle whether the repair is of a point mutation or some grosser chromosomal damage.

There is excellent evidence that irradiation kills bone marrow stem-cells *in vivo* according to the same kinetics as is observed in the cell culture experiments. If we include, as is legitimate, all types of DNA- and chromosome-damage which leave the cell viable and with some mutant character expressed in the descendants, as somatic mutations, the results with cell culture can be regarded as directly relevant to the processes that take place *in vivo*.

The importance of these studies of mammalian cells in culture is to legitimize, as it were, the concept of somatic mutation by showing that it is basically similar to bacterial mutation and, at one remove, of essentially the same qualtiy as germ-line mutation, the accepted raw material of evolution. It is of particular significance that cell culture studies can show that mammalian cells as well as bacteria have well developed DNA repair mechanisms.

Manifestations of somatic mutation

Before moving toward the evidence that somatic mutation plays a major role in ageing, it will be desirable to describe the general characteristics of somatic mutation as manifested in some well studied examples. The fundamental postulate is that mutation occurs in somatic cells in the same way as in the spermatagonia or other cells in the germ line, the only important differences being the absence of the phenomena of meiosis and conjugation before the effect of the mutation can be expressed. In a somatic cell any mutation that can be expressed must be of a dominant or co-dominant character, but if this is the case it will be shown by all descendant cells, subject only to the qualification that, for what can be called inertial reasons, full expression of an established somatic genetic change may not be evident until after two or more cell generations.

As for a germ-line cell, so in somatic cells mutations take place (1) in a single cell, (2) on very rare occasions, and (3) in what we can at present call a wholly random fashion. Any details of what happens when a normal cell is, as it were, tapped on the shoulder and converted into a cell with a new capacity transmissible to its descendants is therefore not accessible to direct study. When we remember that in round figures there are 10^9 cells in any cubic centimetre of living tissue, it is evident enough that the chance of recognizing a change resulting from mutation in the cell primarily involved is vanishingly small. Even if change in the genome renders it non-viable, the cell will be quietly absorbed and vanish. With a few quite exceptional qualifications, there are only two ways by which the existence of somatic mutation can be recognized. The most important is by the appearance of a large uniform population of descendant cells, each cell with the same characteristic differences from the unmutated parent cell. The second, which will be discussed extensively in relation to error catastrophe, is by a progressive degeneration in functional efficiency of a tissue or cell system, resulting from the accumulation of mutational changes. For the present, only the first, i.e. the development of a clone of cells showing some characteristic difference from the parent cell type, need be considered. The changed quality may be recognized by the compact growth of the descendant clone in the form of a tumour or by unusual numbers of relatively normal appearing cells where there should only be few, as in chronic lymphatic leukaemia or some pigmented skin lesions. Sometimes the existence of an aberrant clone of cells can be recognized by the amount or quality of some secretory product. The myeloma proteins, which are essentially large, uniform concentrations of a single type of antibody in the blood, provide the best examples. This uniform 'monoclonal' character of the cells or cell product is a particularly useful criterion to establish the occurrence of a somatic mutation as its origin.

By using this and the other general qualities of somatic mutation, and putting special stress on the monoclonal character of the abnormal cells, one can ascribe to somatic mutation the following physiological and pathological phenomena seen in human beings:

1. The generation of immunological diversity in the stem cells from which immunocytes are derived (see page 65).
2. The results of somatic mutation in embryonic cells shown usually, but not exclusively, in the form of skin blemishes.
3. Benign tumours, such as myomata (fibroids) of the uterus.
4. Malignant and semi-malignant tumours.
5. Autoimmune disease.
6. Another condition that has been ascribed in part to somatic mutation is atherosclerosis, and there may well be others still to be recognized which integrate with the rest to develop the pattern of senescence.

Some short comments may be made on most of these.

Mutation in embryonic cells

It must not be forgotten that mutation can occur in any somatic cell, from the first division of the zygote onwards. Most of the human examples are relatively trivial moles and birth-marks. The most interesting investigation in the field is probably that carried out about twenty years ago on fleece mosaics in Australian sheep. It exemplifies two important principles. The first is the universal one, that a mutation is only demonstrable if the mutant form can proliferate extensively, and second, that a mutation in a certain gene has no effect whatever until the gene attains phenotypic expression. Without going into any detail of the classical work of Fraser and Short[(25)], we may exemplify the two principles by considering one sheep, which showed 50 per cent of the skin with normal fleece, 50 per cent with long, uncrimped wool fibres. The responsible mutation must have occurred either in one of the two cells from the first division of the zygote or (much less probably) from one of the first two descendants of a cell predestined to control the whole skin area. In either case, very large numbers of descendant cells not concerned with the control of wool growth had remained perfectly normal. From the distribution of the long-fibred fleece in vertical stripes or lens-shaped areas one can deduce that approximately half of the cells migrating from the neural crest carried the mutation. At a certain stage of development each of these primary cells developed into a clone whose descendants were responsible for the quality of fleece on one of these irregularly vertical areas. Any other cells which derived from the original mutant must still carry the altered gene but show no evidence of its existence.

The appearance of such a sheep can be mimicked in many respects by using Mintz's technique of blastocyst fusion to produce what she calls an allophenic or tetra-parental mouse[(26)]. The technique, in outline, is to obtain early fertilized ova from the uterus of a mouse of and fertilized by pure strain A and fuse them *in vitro*, each with a similar early embryo of strain B. Using appropriate techniques, the two packets of cells fuse to form a single blastocyst, which is the first stage in the morphological development of the embryo. The blastocyst in which A and B cells in approximately equal numbers appear to be arranged at random is then transferred to the uterus of a foster mother, and if all goes well it is born as a structurally normal mosaic of the two parental strains. If one is coloured and the other white, a proportion of the 'allophenes' will appear as 'zebra mice' with irregularly alternating vertical stripes. In essence, the situation is almost identical to what happens with a somatic mutation in one of the cells of the primary division of the zygote.

One of the most interesting examples of human somatic mutation occurring in embryonic life that I have seen illustrated was a rather lightly pigmented birthmark, elongate oval in shape, and slanting down from the forehead to the eyelids of the left eye. A small portion of what was obviously the end of the birthmark was in the skin of the lower eyelid, separated completely from the other nine-tenths or more. The only possible interpretation was that the clone of mutant melanocytes had spread during early foetal life through the skin covering the future site of the eyes, and with the opening of the palpebral fissure in the fourth or fifth month was divided into two parts[27].

Benign and malignant tumours

The fact that all the cells in an individual tumour are monoclonal in character does not *necessarily* prove that the change in the cell from which it developed was the result of somatic mutation. Nevertheless, if monoclonality is firmly established, any other interpretation requires some ingenious special pleading that is liable to be very unconvincing. In fact most benign and malignant tumours can be shown to be monoclonal in at least a considerable proportion of the cases that can be tested. It is convenient to leave most of the discussion to the chapters dealing with malignant disease, but the important example of benign myomas of the uterus can be dealt with here. It is important, too, to outline the method which in recent years has been applied to determine whether tumours and other focal lesions are monoclonal or not. It depends on the fact that, when females are heterozygous in regard to a sex-linked gene, the two characters are 'allotted' to different cells. All female somatic cells in mammals contain two X chromosomes: one derived paternally from the sperm nucleus, one from the ovum. Only one of the X chromosomes is functional in any cell, the other being rendered functionally inactive in early embryonic life. At that stage some type of decision is made at random in each cell as to whether the paternal or the maternal X chromosome will be inactivated. On the average, 50 per cent of cells make one decision, 50 per cent the other, and once the choice has been made, all descendants of each cell retain the same pattern. The normal tissues of the female are therefore mosaics of two types of cells: one with paternal X chromosome active and expressing qualities carried on it, the other with the maternal X (Figure 6). The enzyme G6PD (glucose-6-phosphate dehydrogenase) can exist in two genetically distinct forms, A and B, the genes involved being carried on the X chromosome. Many African women are heterozygous, so that their body cells, including the smooth muscle cells of the uterus, make up a fine-grained mosaic of A and B. The two forms of the enzyme can be readily identified biochemically in cell extracts. If from a heterozygous AB woman a piece of normal uterus is tested, both A and B enzymes will be found. If, however, tumour tissue of a myoma is examined, it will show either A or B but not both[28]. This rule holds quite regularly and establishes that each myoma arises from a single cell.

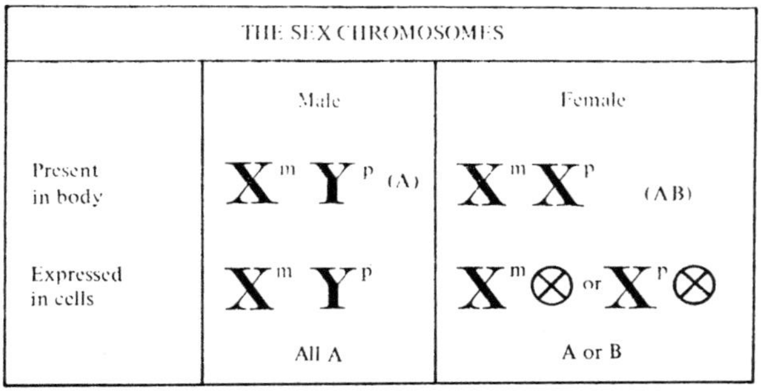

Figure 6 The Lyon phenomenon: inhibition of one X chromosome. When quality A or B is expressed on the X chromosome, it must always be either A or B in the male, which has only one X chromosome. In the female, which has two X chromosomes, one is inactivated in random fashion during embryonic life, so that subsequently the cells make up a mosiac in which approximately equal numbers of cells are A and B, never both. m and p indicate a chromosome derived from maternal or paternal genome respectively

Monoclonality may also be established by the uniformity of a cellular product. Multiple myeloma has already been mentioned as giving rise to a wholly uniform product equivalent to one specific type of antibody molecule; it is also a semi-malignant tumour, very much akin to the leukaemias. The capacity of carcinogenic chemicals (polycyclic hydrocarbons and many other types of compound) to induce malignant tumours in experimental animals is fully established and, like all other tumours, their cells are changed genetically, transmitting the key qualities of their capacity for malignant growth and new antigenic qualities to their descendants. In this sense they have undergone somatic mutation. The interpretation of the role of the chemical carcinogen in the process, however, is one of the most controversial matters in the field of cancer research and can be deferred until Chapter 12. It is relevant to note here, however, that the antigenic diversity amongst such tumours provides incidental evidence that most of them are monoclonal in character.

Autoimmune disease

There are a number of important human diseases which appear to result from a damaging attack by the immune system on normal cells or soluble substances of the body. It is as if the normal taboo has been broken and the body is mistakenly recognizing some of its own constituents as foreign. Among the better known diseases that have been claimed, with some justification, to fall into this category are rheumatoid arthritis, Graves' disease (exophthalmic goitre), pernicious anaemia, and systemic lupus. One of the important indications of autoimmune disease is the presence in the patient's serum of autoantibodies against some body component. It is, however, by no means necessary that the autoantibody that is detectable in the serum is actually causing the signs and symptoms of the disease from which the patient is suffering. It is almost the rule that every clinical disorder of the immune system is a complex one, involving both T- and B-immune systems and partially countered by the body in one way or another. The etiology of autoimmune conditions is a highly controversial topic. If one accepts the clonal selection theory of immunity, it seems axiomatic that autoimmune processes as well as 'normal' immune responses must be concordant with it. I have recently re-examined the 'forbidden clone' hypothesis[29, 30], which has now been current for some fifteen years, and find no reason to modify its main features. It can be stated in outline as follows:

> An autoimmune disease is the result of the emergence of one or more clones of immunocytes which in addition to a certain immune pattern directed against self-components are resistant to the standard controls which eliminate or inhibit immunocytes reactive against self-substance in normal animals. They are 'forbidden clones' in virtue or two or more somatic mutations that have occurred in their ancestral somatic cell line.

We are still far from a detailed interpretation of autoimmune disease, and in addition to the appearance of forbidden clones there are complex interactions of various sorts with other aspects of the immune system. Apart from noting that in three types of autoimmune haemolytic anaemia monoclonality can be demonstrated, further discussion can be left for a later chapter.

Atherosclerosis

A major role in the vascular pathology of people beyond middle life is ascribed to atherosclerosis, but there has been no clear understanding of how the characteristic plaques in the intima of the aorta and medium-sized arteries arise. This makes the claim by Benditt and Benditt[31], in mid-1973, that the cells in individual atheromatous plaques are monoclonal of special significance.

There are so many implications of this finding, if it can be confirmed, that it seems justifiable to leave its full discussion for a separate chapter. Here it need only be said that the investigation was made on autopsy material from negro women heterozygous for the A and B forms of the enzyme G6PD. The techniques were similar to those used in establishing the monoclonal character of uterine myomata and were carried out in the same medical school. The results appear clear cut; the normal intima contains both A and B enzymes; pieces from early discrete lesions are either A or B, about a third are sharply A or B, the others all show a great predominance of one with traces of the other, except for one or two with both in more or less equivalent quantity. These deviations from strict monoclonality are only to be expected when one considers the complexity of the tissue concerned. The essential part played by the blood levels of cholesterol and other lipids in the development of atherosclerosis, in addition to any initiating somatic mutation, must of course be kept firmly in mind.

PART 2

Physiology and Pathology of Ageing

CHAPTER 6

THE MANIFESTATIONS OF AGEING

The pattern of old age in man, at least as it manifests itself in our own particular social environment, is known to everyone. Many will have noticed how similar the process is in a dog or a horse. That general background is sufficient for most purposes, but at the risk of occasionally underlining the obvious it is clearly desirable to include a chapter on those segments of the manifestations of ageing which most require to be covered in a theoretical inquiry. It will be influenced largely by Comfort's book(32) and by my special interest in immunity and cancer as related to age.

Information about the facts of ageing in man comes mostly from vital statistics and clinical studies with, nowadays, extensive collections of surveys of what may be relevant data from normal populations. For the main domestic animals a certain amount of information can be gleaned from stud books and there is much casual and anecdotal knowledge, particularly about instances of exceptional longevity, from breeders. In addition, we have numerous laboratory studies of ageing and its parameters in chosen strains of mice, rats or hamsters. In general, my account will concentrate on human manifestations, and make reference to the experimental work on rodents where necessary. No reference will be made to invertebrates and very little to any other class of vertebrates than the mammals.

The time of death

The most important correlate of ageing is death. An increasing vulnerability to potentially lethal impacts from trauma, infection, or internal accident is obviously associated with age. A graph published by Comfort, showing that the age distribution of pedestrians killed on the roads is closely parallel to that of all deaths, is revealing. Deaths from infections in which past immunization by natural or artificial means is absent or irrelevant show a similar regularity in the increase of mortality with age. This is shown when some exotic infectious disease invades a community which has never previously experienced the infection, but it is shown just as clearly for relatively non-specific infections with short-lasting immunity of respiratory tract or bowel (Figure 7).

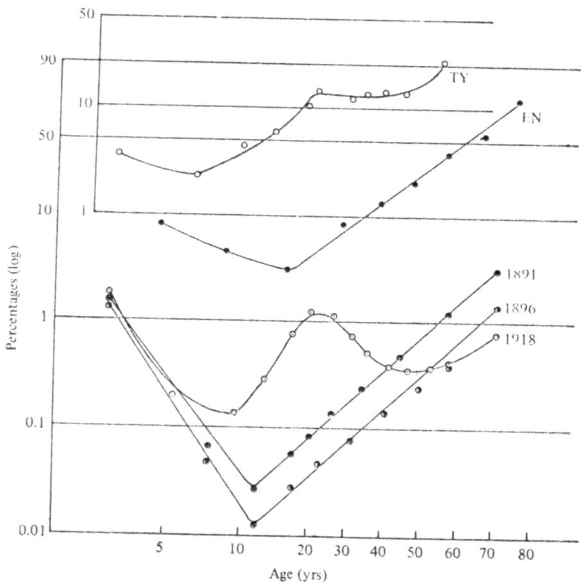

Figure 7 Infectious disease curves. To show increased mortality with age from (*a*) specific conditions to which the individuals are non-immune: the example shows fatality rates for typhoid fever, Western Australia (TY) and St Louis encephalitis (EN) (1933). The typhoid scale is inset. (*b*) Infections of a non-specific character: the example shows infections in two 'influenza' years (1891 and 1918) and a 'non-influenza' year (1896). (Note. The time-scale changes from logarithmic to linear at twenty-five years.)

Influenza epidemics provide the most conspicuous examples. Whenever the weekly death records of a sizable city show for a few weeks in winter a sharp rise above the standard level, one can be almost certain that an epidemic of influenza A has been responsible. Most of these excess deaths will be found to involve people over sixty, and the highest incidence will be on the very old and those with some form of chronic illness. In the days when tuberculosis was a major cause of death the yearly curve of mortality from the disease could be expected to show a sharp rise in an influenza year, to be followed next year by a corresponding low. More than one weakness may play a part in the fatal outcome, but both old age and chronic tuberculosis are associated with depressed immune responses and it is simplest and probably correct to ascribe death to a failure of the immune reactions that were called for. With the development of treatment with antibiotics, deaths from infection have

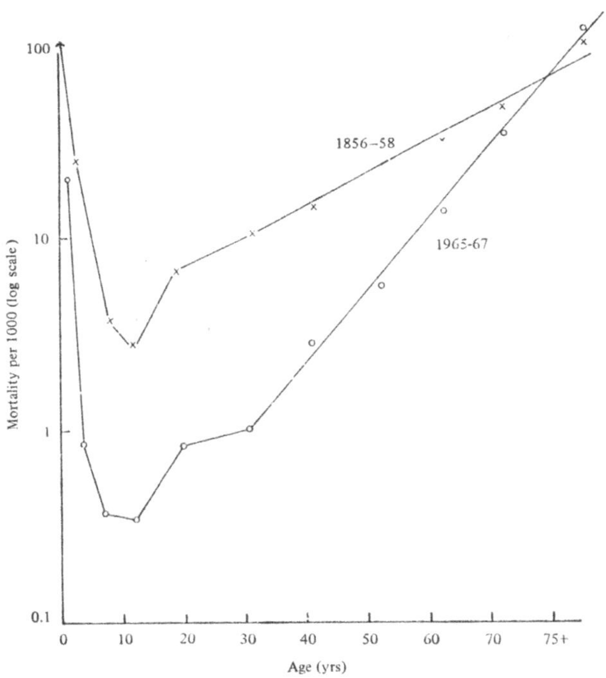

Figure 8 The age-specific mortality in Victoria (Australia) for 1856–1858 and 1965–1967 to show the approximate straight line from 20–30 onwards when plotted in semi-logarithmic fashion. (Gompertz curve)

diminished greatly and mortality curves have changed their shape but not their general quality. The regularity of the relationship between age and death can best be seen when age-specific death rates are plotted on a logarithmic scale against age to give the conventional Gompertz curve. For age-specific mortality figures it is conventional to work with five-year age groups—0–4, 5–9, and so on—and to record deaths per thousand per annum in each group. For any reasonably stable population the Gompertz curve approximates closely to a straight line from the age of twenty onwards.

In Figure 8 I have plotted the age-specific mortality curves for the State of Victoria in 1858–1860 and in 1967 as an example of the changes that a hundred years will show in almost any relatively advanced part of the world. In the mid-nineteenth century deaths before maturity were vastly more numerous than in our present epoch. Most were due to infections of various types. From around thirty onwards, however, both lines are approximately straight and reach almost the same point at seventy and over. It is interesting, and to be expected, that the survivors in 1860 who had reached seventy years had a slightly better mortality record than their contemporaries today. The important, the defining, feature of the line is its slope, essentially indicating the size of a constant annual increase in the probability of dying. This constant is often referred to as 'the force of mortality' acting on the population. In a sense every death has some element of the accidental, but no matter how heavy or how light is the lethal impact of the environment, the direct relationship of age and death is always evident.

The signs of ageing

The first sign of ageing to become obvious to others is greying of the hair. The timing of the change as measured by the first recognition of grey hairs and by the completion of the change to a head of white hair varies greatly from person to person. Over a whole population, however, stochastic regularities emerge and both the beginning and the end of the process show a smooth relationship with age[33, 34]. Greying is essentially an increase in the number of individual hairs in which melanocytes fail to develop during the growth of the hair[35]. Each individual hair has limited life and after it has fallen out the hair bulb, including the pigment-producing melanocytes, needs to be reconstructed. If after a pigmented hair has been lost the bulb does not receive melanocytes, the resulting hair is white, and a further step in the process of greying has been taken. Greying with age is seen in dogs and other mammals and an accelerated form is seen in most of the breeds of horses that are grey or white at maturity. The Lipizzaners of the Spanish Riding School in Vienna usually develop a pure white coat between the ages of seven and ten years. In these and in 'white horses' generally, the patchy development of white areas, dappling, is characteristic of the intermediate stage between the black or brown of the young animal and the white of maturity. It is of interest that white horses retain a pigmented skin and are prone to pigmented tumours (melanomas).

In the majority of old people irregular mottling of the skin is present in the areas normally exposed to sunlight, particularly on the backs of the hands. Most of the mottling is due to irregular patches of brown pigment and occasional areas of depigmentation, but areas of thickened epidermis, hypekeratoses, also play a part.

Reduction in the amount of collagen in the tissues and a steady deterioration in its functional quality are regularly associated with ageing in man and experimental mammals. These changes are largely responsible for the physical frailty of old persons. The effects of the diminution in amount and loss of strength and elasticity of collagen with age are seen chiefly in the thinning and wrinkling of the skin and in the fragility of the bones. Collagen fibres form an essential tensile support in bone, and its atrophy, associated with resorption of calcium, is responsible for one of the commonest mishaps of old age, fracture of the neck of the femur.

Post-mortem examination of old people shows an increasing brown pigmentation of the heart due to a protein-containing pigment, lipofuscin[36]. Similar 'age-pigment' accumulates in a variety of organs and in most species studied. Quantitative studies show a fairly steady accumulation through life, but a wide scatter of individual values.

Age-related changes in many physiological functions in man have been examined, including basal metabolic rate, vital capacity, and renal plasma flow. All show a more or less linear decline with age[37]. Everyone is aware of the differences in 'physical fitness' that can be seen in individuals of the same chronological age. It is common to think of these as pointers to the potential longevity of the individual and often enough expectations are fulfilled. Obviously, however, some more quantitative approach to the prediction of longevity and the quality of old age is needed, and one of the important tasks for gerontological research is to define a series of measurable characteristics of men and women that can serve as indices of the progress of ageing. One can be certain that if several are measured in the same individual not all of them will give the same answer, but, as Comfort has pointed out[38], such a collection of what can be called parameters of ageing would help immensely in assessing the extent to which the process of ageing is influenced by environmental factors from childhood onward.

Age-associated disease

In addition to the deaths that can be ascribed to an increasing vulnerability to potentially lethal factors in the environment, we have a range of age-associated deaths in which the predominant etiological component seems to be intrinsic to the indvidual. If the concept of age-associated disease is to be made precise, it must be based on an adequate knowledge of the age-specific incidence of the disease, which for commonly lethal conditions is most often derived from the recorded age at death. Morbidity surveys of statistically acceptable samples of populations have provided similar information for some common non-lethal conditions, such as chronic arthritis. For those who are not specialists in mathematical statistics the most convenient way of presenting the data is to determine for each five-year age group the number of cases per 10 000 of the population at risk and plot this as incidence against age. For most purposes it is convenient to use logarithmic scales for both incidence and age. It has been known, ever since reasonably accurate records of mortality with a stated cause of death have been available, that death from 'all cancers' and from most of the common cancers of specific sites, when plotted in this fashion, gave an upward sloping straight line with a slope of 5 or 6. Typical examples of such graphs will be seen in Figures 9 and 15. Similar straight lines rising to the end of life are also seen for such conditions as death from coronary disease or cerebrovascular disease and for the incidence of osteoarthritis, fracture of the neck of the femur, or grey hair. For our purposes the age-associated diseases are those that show this type of age-specific incidence graph, approximating a straight line over the significant period from about twenty-five to seventy-five and showing a steepness of at least 4.

One or two comments on the significance of this definition of age-associated disease may be offered:

1. An essential feature is that the curve extends downward to at least twenty-five or thirty, i.e. that deaths from typical age-associated diseases

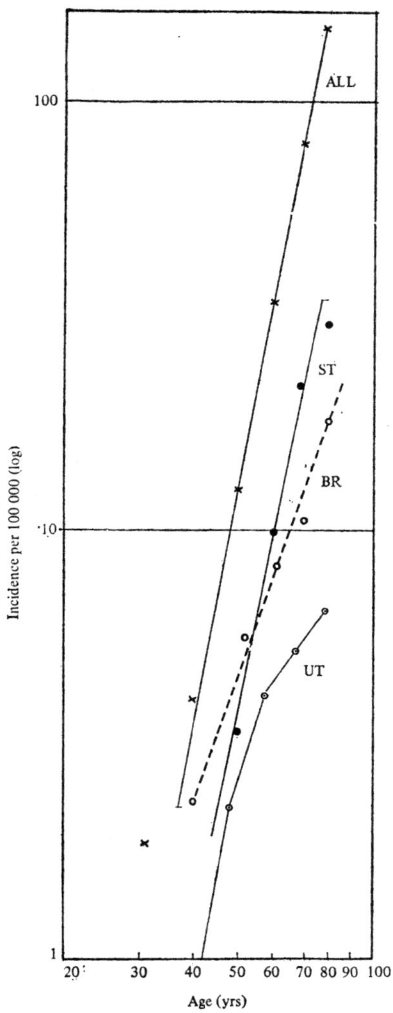

Figure 9 The age-specific incidence of cancer mortality. Incidence per 100 000 at risk is shown on a logarithmic scale, as are ages from 20 to 100. ALL = All cancers in males; ST = Cancer of stomach in males; BR = Cancer of breast in females; UT = Cancer of uterus

occur in young adult life. It is the regular, continuing increase with age that defines their nature.

2. When numbers of subjects become small over seventy-five, the curve often deviates from a straight line for such causes as increasing uncertainty of diagnosis, a cohort effect when some significant etiological factor has been changing over the life-time of elderly people, or the emergence of a small group of genetically long-lived individuals.

3. It will be remembered that the Gompertz curve for overall mortality rises regularly with age but approaches more closely to a straight line when plotted semi-logarithmically, i.e. incidence on a logarithmic scale, age on a linear one, than with both scales logarithmic. This holds, too, for deaths from respiratory infections and for environmental causes generally, acting presumably on a basis of vulnerability increasing with age.

The straight line curve on a double log plot, according to Doll[39], provides an inadequate base on which to build a theory of cancer *ab initio*, but, equally, no suggested mechanism that fails to lead to this relationship can possibly be valid. Fully admitting mathematical incompetence, I have found it useful to assume (*a*) that the Gompertz curve approaching a straight line on a semi-log plot is based on increasing vulnerability to environmental impact and (*b*) that the straight line on a double log plot indicates some combination of self-activating processes of intrinsic origin which include, particularly, multi-stage episodes such as sequential somatic mutation and proliferation of potentially pathogenic cells. Most deaths nowadays in the old result from degeneration and secondary changes in some part of the cardiovascular system. That group includes not only ischaemic heart disease (heart attacks, coronary obstruction) and congestive heart failure, but also arteriosclerosis, aneurysms, and cerebral vascular catastrophes (strokes). Taken together, these make up about 60 per cent of the stated causes of death in people over sixty-five. Cancer of all types is responsible for 16 to 20 per cent.

In addition to lethal conditions there are a number of chronic diseases and disabilities that are equally characteristic of old age. Perhaps the most striking group of disabilities involves the joints; proverbially the old man hobbles with a stick. Conventionally, the two main forms of joint disease and disability are differentiated as rheumatoid arthritis and osteoarthritis, and classical examples of the two diseases are completely distinct.

Rheumatoid arthritis tends to involve the hands, wrists and feet, and often shows severe exacerbations with marked subacute inflammation around the affected joints. About 30 per cent of patients, particularly those with severe symptoms, show a characteristic autoantibody, 'rheumatoid factor', in the blood. This reacts with immunoglobulin and there is presumptive evidence that interaction of immunoglobulin as antigen with rheumatoid factor, which can be thought of as immunoglobulin in autoantibody guise, is responsible for much of the damage to the joint lining. Osteoarthritis is a more slowly developing condition, usually of the weight-bearing joints, and is generally regarded as a purely degenerative process. Both rheumatoid arthritis and osteoarthritis become increasingy prevalent with age and it is stated that in the United States as many as 85 per cent of people over seventy shows signs of osteoarthritis, with moderate to serious disability in nearly half of them. Burch[40], who has made extensive mathematical analysis of the age incidence of chronic disease, deduces that there is no proportion of human beings who are genetically insusceptible to either disease. The two diseases as diagnosed show quite distinct age-incidence patterns and, in the case of rheumatoid arthritis, about twice as many affected women as men. Burch considers that the incidence of each can be fitted to an appropriate stochastic curve, indicating that a series of interrelated random processes is responsible in each disease for the emergence of the diagnosable syndrome (Figure 10).

Both diseases are so common that if they have quite distinct etiologies one would expect to find large numbers of individuals with both. The possibility that all chronic joint conditions have degenerative, inflammatory, reparative, and autoimmune processes manifested in varying mixtures and that all are age-associated seems as likely as any other interpretation.

Rheumatoid arthritis may or may not be wholly a manifestation of autoimmune disease, but there are certainly autoimmune processes demonstrably involved in more than half the cases. Rather similar statements can be made about late onset diabetes, pernicious anaemia, and a variety of less well known conditions. By no means all autoimmune diseases are age-associated in this fashion. Burch's view is that the autoimmune conditions which show a peak of incidence before middle age, like systemic lupus erythematosus (SLE) and Graves' disease of the thyroid (exophthalmic goitre), occur only in individuals with a genetic predisposition to the disease. Where such a potentiality to develop an autoimmune disease exists, the probability that any susceptible individual not yet involved will develop the disease steadily increases with age. The

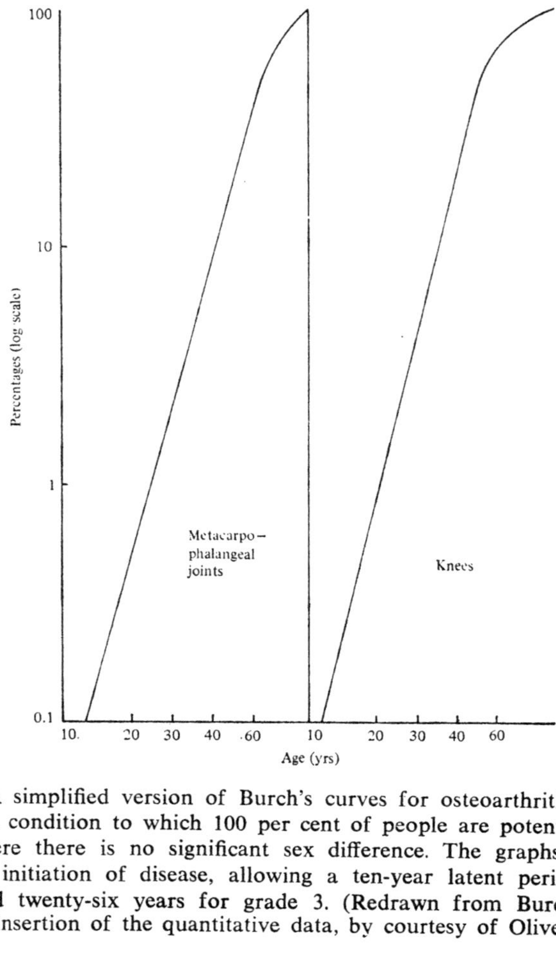

Figure 10 A simplified version of Burch's curves for osteoarthritis. This is an example of a condition to which 100 per cent of people are potentially susceptible and where there is no significant sex difference. The graphs are for the incidence of initiation of disease, allowing a ten-year latent period for grade 2 lesions and twenty-six years for grade 3. (Redrawn from Burch[40] (Figure 4.3) without insertion of the quantitative data, by courtesy of Oliver and Boyd.)

rapid disappearance of new cases after a certain age merely means that the susceptibles have been used up.

Autoimmunity, with that reservation, is an age-associated disease and will be discussed more extensively at a later stage.

Other disabilities of old age include cataract and other senile changes in the eye, deafness, and a wide range of signs of cerebral degeneration and dysfunction, from minor loss of short-term memory to gross senile psychoses and degeneration. In general, there is no measurable aspect of bodily function which fails to show some quantitative loss of efficiency with age. Wisdom and experience may mask the evidence of that inefficiency for a long time, but it will always emerge. In many ways the major difficulty in interpreting senescence is to assess what interactions are concerned in producing the various inefficiencies that are observed. In particular, there is always likely to be controversy as to how far changes in the immune system and in the effectiveness of the cardiovascular supply of blood to the tissues are primarily responsible for many of the aspects of ageing.

On the whole, not a great deal that is relevant to human ageing and its associated diseases has been learnt from animal studies, and a brief account will be sufficient.

In the species of laboratory animals that have been used for detailed studies of ageing the pathological findings in those dying or terminally ill generally resemble what is seen in man[41, 42] In rats, myocardial degeneration and chronic glomerulonephritis reach nearly 100 per cent by three years and periarteritis 50 per cent. Malignant and semi-malignant tumours increase with age. Mice strains can vary greatly in regard to average lifespan, but the short-lived ones usually die from some characteristic disease: AKR from leukaemia, and the NZB/NZW hybrid from autoimmune kidney disease. In general, when mice or rats have their lifespan shortened by irradiation, the age-associated diseases, including tumours, occur correspondingly earlier (with occasional discrepancies), while in rats, whose lifespan is prolonged by restriction of diet after weaning, the onset of tumours and degenerative disease is delayed correspondingly. Such findings point strongly to a common basis for ageing and for most age-associated diseases.

CHAPTER 7

AGEING: THE SOMATIC MUTATIONAL APPROACH

The whole process of evolution demands that all the individuals of one generation must die to make way for the generation that succeeds them, but there is no special evolutionary demand that death should be led up to by a period of senescence analogous to what we find in ourselves. There may be nothing whatever in common in the means by which death comes to the mayfly, the salmon after spawning, and the man over sixty-five. There are many animal species, notably most of the smaller birds, where mortality from predators is so high that there is no significant opportunity for senescence to have any meaning for evolution. Even if, as is usual, we confine our interest to man and the other mammals, there are several different aspects that call for investigation, and virtually every investigator finds one more interesting than the others. However, probably all modern workers will accept that somatic mutation plays a considerable part, and the recent developments that interest me chiefly all seem to point in that direction. They include particularly the discovery of the Hayflick limit[(43)], its establishment for immunocyte clones *in vivo* by Williamson and Askonas[(44)], and the hints that the limit is reached by the process called 'error catastrophe' by Orgel[(45)]. All of these phenomena are intimately concerned with somatic mutation. Taken together, they provide the best central theme for discussion as a basis of senescence, but this does not at all exclude the existence of other factors independently associated with ageing. Everything in this chapter has reference to ways in which somatic mutation can be used in developing an interpretation of the ageing process. Pride of place is given to the Hayflick-Orgel approach, but the two other approaches, by Burch and Curtis respectively, are also considered.

The significance of the Hayflick limit

The Hayflick limit is a concept derived from experiments by Hayflick[43] on the serial culture of fibroblasts from human embryo lungs. Under optimal cultural conditions these cells continue to proliferate during successive transfer to new medium over long periods and retain their characteristic diploid number of 46 chromosomes. As the cultures approach 50 cell generations from the time of their establishment, mitosis becomes irregular and the cells eventually cease to proliferate. Only if a change involving chromosome number and regularity occurs will a human or a mouse cell line continue growing indefinitely. For normal non-malignant diploid cells, 50 ± 14 generations is the limit, a limit now usually referred to by the name of the cytologist who discovered it.

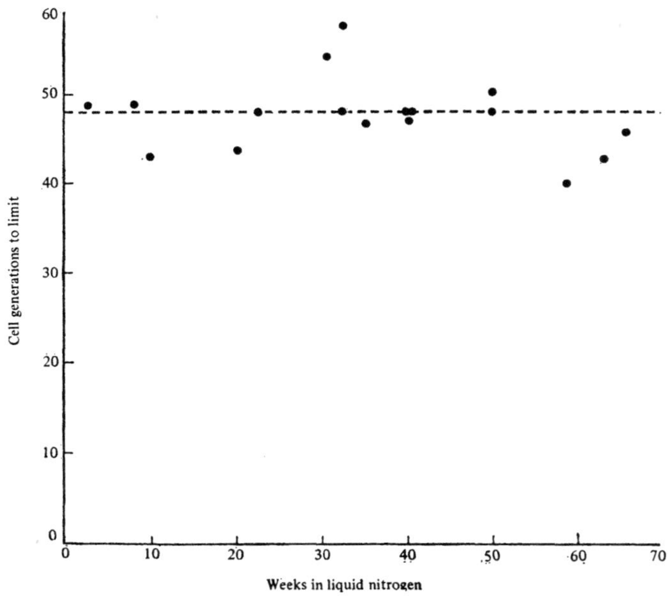

Figure 11 The Hayflick limit. In this experiment by Hayflick the number of cell generations before proliferation failed (Phase III) is shown for seventeen samples of the same human diploid cell culture stored in liquid nitrogen. Average value = forty-seven generations

At an early stage Hayflick suggested that this type of limitation on continued somatic cell mutation might be basic to the determination of lifespan in mammals. The suggestion has had a mixed reception, largely because of doubts as to whether results in cell culture could be taken as indicating that similar limitations to growth held *in vivo*. Franks[(46)] and Walford[(47)] both looked to technical inadequacies in cell culture methods as the most likely reason for the eventual failure of mitosis in diploid somatic cells. It is not easy to devise ways of showing what happens *in vivo* in this respect, and the results that have been published are inconclusive[(48)], except for recent immunological work, to be described later.

On the positive side, the most interesting contribution is that of Martin *et al.*[(49)], who studied fibroblast cultures from the skin of donors of all ages. They found a fairly consistent negative regression of growth potential on age of donor, with an average limit of 42 cell generations in children under ten, falling steadily with age to 28 in the age group eighty to ninety. Anomalously low values for donors with genetic abnormalities associated with accelerated ageing were also found in this investigation, but it is convenient to leave their discussion to a later stage. On the whole, there is probably a majority opinion that the Hayflick limit measures an important biological quality of somatic cells which is significant for the interpretation of ageing.

The currently popular suggestion as to why mitosis fails as the Hayflick limit is approached was advanced in 1963. The basic idea was probably derived from earlier suggestions by Wulff *et al.*[(50)], but took its current form in Orgel's concept of error catastrophe[(45)]. In essence, the idea is that somatic mutation, involving an enzyme critically concerned in the maintenance of DNA integrity (on successive duplication) or in one of the informational transfers by which protein is synthesized, will automatically result in errors involving a progressively wider range of enzymes, so that at a certain point there is an error catastrophe which will mean a final breakdown in the viability of the cell. Orgel took the widely accepted view that the significant somatic mutations were those occurring in non-dividing (post-mitotic) cells. In these, the most significant point at which error accumulation could be initiated would be at the transcription stage, as a result of structural change in RNA polymerase or one of the other enzymes concerned. A destructive end result could be initiated by inefficiency in any enzyme that plays a part in assuring fidelity in synthesis of primary polypeptide chains, and for most purposes the precise enzyme or group of enzymes concerned is immaterial.

Evidence in favour of the general concept has been published from several laboratories, using experiments which demonstrated the appearance of abnormal enzymes in cell cultures approaching the Hayflick limit. A discusion of these results can be deferred to Chapter 11. Another important point that can only be mentioned and set aside for later consideration is the difficulty of accounting for the *absence* of such a process of cumulative error in cells which have changed from the diploid phase or become malignant.

What is more important at this stage is to look for evidence that the Hayflick limit is relevant within the body. There are very obvious difficulties here. Living cells are always the descendants of other cells, but in the complexities of embryonic development and post-natal growth it is very difficult to decipher more than an outline of the sequence by which a definitive cell type is developed from primitive, undifferentiated embryonic cells and ultimately from the fertilised ovum, the single-cell zygote. We know, too, that there are many important cell types that are constantly dying and being disposed of one way or another. Every day 1 per cent of our red blood cells are removed, mostly in the spleen, and are being replaced by new cells from the bone marrow. The white cells of the blood are used up and replaced even more rapidly; so too are the epithelial cells of the skin and of the mucous membranes that line the respiratory and gastrointestinal tract. In a less conspicuous fashion there is a constant turnover of cells in most of the other tissues of the body. The major exceptions are the cells of the nervous system and of the muscles which at least in adult life are not replaced.

Obviously each type of cell has its own particular line of descent from the zygote, and we can be sure that there are landmarks along the road where successive levels of differentiation take place. At a certain point, too, in some lines we reach a stage at which multiplication ceases, the cell is fully differentiated and takes on its definitive function. Once that stage is reached it may persist, as in the central nervous system, for the life of the animal, or, depending on its type and the occurrence of accident, for any lesser period. With complete knowledge we might be able to say how many cell generations intervened between all those changes. The cell line that we shall be specially interested in is that which leads to the cells concerned with immunity: the lymphocyte and the plasma cell. Our knowledge of that sequence is very far from complete, but we know enough to allow us to use the lymphocyte line as an example of the general pattern of cell behaviour in lines with continuing clonal proliferation.

The lymphocyte (immunocyte) series

In a general sketch of the process of lymphoid cell differentiation we may start with the early divisions of the fertilised ovum to form after about a dozen cell generations a blastula in which there is the first sign that cells are becoming differentiated towards eventual function. Somewhere about this point we can probably assume that a certain cell is predestined to become a blood cell and not a skin cell or a nerve cell. A number of choices, however, are still open to it. Depending on circumstance, it may become a red cell, platelet, lymphocyte, monocyte, or granulocyte. At this stage it may be called a stem cell, in the sense that from its continued multiplication any of these forms may eventually arise. We can regard this stem cell as the first step in the series.

The stem cell arises in or soon moves to a suitable organ where it can persist and multiply. In the case of the blood stem cells in vertebrates, the organ concerned changes as the embryo develops, from the yolk sac to the liver and spleen, and, after birth or hatching, to the red bone marrow in ribs, vertebrae, and the ends of the long bones of the limbs. At the next step the stem cell makes the 'decision' as to which type of blood cell it will become; in the line we are following, a lymphocyte and not a red cell or a granulocyte. Most likely, the direction of the change depends on the action on the stem cell of certain hormones, of which the best known is erythropoietin. Effective contact of a stem cell with erythropoietin acts as a trigger which sets the cell along the process of differentiation that leads to the red blood cell. The corresponding hormone for the lymphocyte is not so clearly known. Current opinion is that there may be two, one produced in the thymus which gives rise to T-lymphocytes (short for thymus-dependent lymphocytes), and the other 'somewhere else'. In chickens, the second site is a curious organ, the bursa of Fabricius which develops as a pouch-like outgrowth from the cloaca, and retains an opening into the bowel lumen. During embryonic life it accumulates epithelial and lymphoid cells to form something that histologically is reminiscent of the human tonsil at the opposite end of the alimentary canal. It atrophies at sexual maturity in both sexes. In man and mammals generally, a similar function may devolve on some of the numerous types of cell in the bone marrow. In any case a second major group, the B-lymphocytes (thymus-independent lymphocytes—the ones that produce circulating antibody) develop and cooperate with T-lymphocytes in immunity.

Probably just as soon as the blood line stem cell came into being a process was initiated which would define the character of the antibodies that its descendants would eventually produce. This still rather mysterious process, often spoken of as the generation of diversity in immune pattern, is essential to provide the variety of immune response that will be needed. Both sorts of lymphocyte produce antibody, but in the T-cells only enough is produced to be built into the cell surface as receptors by which the cell can recognize a foreign material, an antigen, with which it can react. The B-cells also carry antibody receptors, but in addition they are liable to synthesize large amounts of antibody and liberate it into the blood. In the process they often take on the form of a plasma cell, which can be looked on as a cell specialised for the synthesis and liberation of large amounts of its specific antibody.

At a later stage we shall be very largely concerned with the thymus and the T-lymphocytes that arise from it, but in the present context the B-cells better illustrate the process of progressive differentiation. At an early stage B-lymphocytes develop specific antibody-type receptors on the cell surface and are known as antigen-reactive cells (ARCs). When such a cell meets an antigen with which its receptor can react, proliferation begins, and, subject to a number of complications which may be neglected, two sorts of cell arise: 'memory cells', and antibody-producing plasma cells. Memory cells are essentially ARCs with more receptors and a more active proliferative response to contact with antigen. Their offspring also include both memory cells and antibody producers. Plasma cells can be regarded as a final stage; at most, they may multiply for 6 to 8 cell generations, then they become quiescent but may persist for weeks.

That account is oversimplified, even in terms of present knowledge, and will undoubtedly be expressed very differently in twenty years' time. Its object is simply to provide a background for discussion of the cell populations whose fate seems to be so closely tied in with the ageing process. The Hayflick limit has been studied in detail only in human fibroblast cell cultures, and if it is to be applied to lymphocytes (immunocytes) in order to explain the atrophy of the immune system with age, some experimental justification is needed. Fortunately this has recently become available with the publication of some important experiments by Williamson and Askonas[44].

They worked with mice, mice which had been converted almost into passive test tubes, in which their own antibody-producing cells could not grow but where immune cells from a normal mouse could proliferate and produce antibody. Such mice can be produced by giving them a heavy dose of X-rays and then 'saving' them by an injection of cells from a normal mouse. Into these test tube mice the experimenters injected cells from normal mice which had been immunized with a suitable well defined antigen. By some ingenious manipulations which need not be detailed they obtained some mice in which a single clone of antibody-producing cells became established, i.e. they were all descendants of a single immune cell and therefore produced a recognizably uniform type of antibody. This provided a unique opportunity to follow what happened in a single line of cells, since the cells identified themselves automatically by producing this particular sort of antibody.

As soon as the first 'test tube mouse' was shown to be actively producing antibody it was killed, and spleen cells, which included B-lymphocytes, mostly memory cells, as well as some antibody producers, were tranferred from it to another irradiated mouse with a small dose of antigen to stimulate some of the memory cells. This sort of transfer was then continued. It worked regularly for seven transfers and failed consistently on the eighth. The only reason that could be given was that there was a limit to the number of cell generations that any single clone of cells could encompass. Appropriate calculations indicated that the limiting number of generations was close to what Hayflick found with human cell cultures.

I have no doubt that sooner or later a new generation of investigators will find other ways of following clones of cells through the body, but at the present time this work on immune lymphocytes is unique. Nevertheless, it was done by experienced and critical investigators, and most immunologists would probably agree that it has been one of the most important immunological advances of the 1970s. It has, too, the great advantage of involving the sort of cells, immune lymphocytes—immunocytes is a convenient name for them—that seem to play a major part in the process of ageing. This is the main reason for this diversion into immunology. It could mean that the Hayflick limit is not something that is relevant only to cell cultures in the laboratory. One must not, however, assume that cumulative somatic mutation of the type leading to an error catastrophe will always result in conditions allowing a definable Hayflick limit. If the process develops slowly and there is a strong differential in rate of proliferation favouring unmutated cells as against those beginning to accumulate mutations, losses by error catastrophe might never be demonstrable. It must also be remembered that large numbers of cell lines actively proliferating during immaturity cease to multiply according to their genetic programme and function as post-mitotics.

Gerontologists unsympathetic to the use of the Hayflick limit as a model for the ageing process have raised two other difficulties. Almost any piece of human tissue that is given the opportunity will produce a cell culture in which the uniform cells that proliferate are fibroblast type. It is, however, by no means sure that these are derived from cells which would be identified as fibroblasts in standard tissue sections. This can hardly be regarded as a reason for not accepting a form of behaviour common to all such cultures as have been studied. A second objection is the possibility that the 'limit' is no more than some inadequacy of the culture medium. Again, this does not invalidate the results of Hayflick-type experiments done under standard conditions, particularly in those, to be discussed later, where cell cultures from genetically abnormal individuals are compared with normal cultures.

Possibly the real importance of the Hayflick limit is the indication that when the experimental conditions are appropriate the limit provides a clear indication that Orgel's postulated error catastrophe *can* occur. This justifies the use of the hypothesis of cumulative somatic errors in clonally proliferating lines *in vivo* to account for diminishing cell numbers and declining efficiency, even if nothing as clear cut as a Hayflick limit is evident.

The consequences of cumulative error in somatic cells will show quite other characteristics in post-mitotic cell population, but again it will lead to a progressive loss (fall-out) of functioning cells, usually with atrophy of the tissue.

As soon as one starts thinking about some of the more specific types of degenerative disease arising in middle life or later, one is inevitably led to consider whether the process at work may not represent an accelerated ageing in one particular system. For many decades it has been part of the conventional wisdom that different systems aged at different speeds. One man was as old as his arteries, another was bound to succumb to the first influenza virus to reach him, and a third lapsed into dementia. Basically this point of view is almost certainly correct and would fit naturally into our present hypothesis, but in so doing would call for an additional postulate. It would demand that there are genes coding individually for DNA polymerases or other key enzymes specific for one or a limited range of cell types. The pattern of a man's ageing would then depend on the distribution of error-proneness over his whole repertoire of key enzymes. With any exceptional concentration of infidelity on a single gene and enzyme, the result will present as a genetic disease, usually an autosomal dominant condition with variable penetrance and a characteristic age-specific incidence curve.

The mathematical approach

For every morbid condition that has accepted diagnostic criteria it is possible in principle to state the age at which the affected individual first presented diagnostic symptoms of the condition, the proportion of people found to be suffering from it, from an adequate sampling of a community and their ages, and finally the numbers and age at death of persons certified as dying from the disease. Any of those sets of data can provide material for analysis of the age-specific incidence of the condition. For obvious reasons the certified cause of deaths provides the most easily accessible material and for many years it has been known that the age patterns of mortality differed greatly, and in general reproducibly, from one disease to another. The distributions are susceptible to mathematical analysis and it is self-evident that if the plotted curves of age incidence for a given disease are similar in several distinct populations, this is a reproducible phenomenon that calls for investigation. More importantly, any interpretation of the etiology and pathogenesis of the disease must be in a form compatible with the observed influence of age. This rather specialized area of epidemiology in the widest sense has been dominated over the last dozen years by the work of P. R. J. Burch[(40)]. Burch's earlier work was concerned with the factors that could be concerned in the characteristic age patterns of malignant disease. My development of the forbidden clone hypothesis of autoimmune disease had sufficient analogies with his approach to malignant disease for Burch to use that hypothesis in interpreting the age-specific incidence of rheumatoid arthritis. Subsequently he has extended and elaborated his approach to cover all the better documented type of chronic and degenerative disease and to develop a general interpretation of ageing. His technique in outline is to prepare curves of age incidence on a double-log plot and to find an appropriate mathematical (stochastic) equation which will fit the curves.

He has summarized the basis of his equations as being the following simple biological model:

1. In autoimmune (or autoaggressive) disease, spontaneous somatic gene mutations are needed to initiate the disease.

2. Throughout life, gene instability follows a law of the same form as that of radioactive decay.

3. Multiple somatic mutations may occur in a single cell (or in a single cell line sequentially to reach a single cell in which all the necessary changes have been accumulated), but in other circumstances n cells may be each subject to a different somatic mutation.

It is understood that the equations are based on the two assumptions that the population of cells susceptible to mutation remains constant and that on the average a cell that is lost is replaced by another cell of the same type, normal or mutant. Burch, however, also accepts a low level of probability that one or more intermediate stages of clonal growth might occur in between random events.

On these assumptions the application of mathematical statistics provides a series of stochastic models which, with appropriate constants, give impressive fits with sex and age-specific graphs of incidence. The basic equations are age-specific prevalence

$$P^t = S\ 1 - \exp(-kt)^n \tag{1}$$

and

$$P^t = S\ 1 - \exp(-kt^r) \tag{2}$$

where n = the number of cells in which a single somatic mutation is necessary and r = the number of mutations in a single cell for the second type of initiation, S is the fraction of the population at birth this is genetically susceptible to the disease, $K = Lm$ in (1) where L is the number of cells at risk and m the mutation rate, $K = Lm^r$ in (2).

According to Burch, 'ageing consists in the main of a very large number of specific autoaggresive disorders'. He excludes malignant disease from this category. There are wide variations in the proportion S who are susceptible to the different autoaggressive diseases, and the genetic factors responsible may be monogenic or polygenic.

To take an example of a disease that is a very frequent cause of death in the elderly, his graph for death from coronary disease (1968, page 44) shows a steep, almost straight, line curve which he interprets as indicating that three conditions hold:

A All individuals are genetically susceptible.
B $r = 6$, i.e. 6 sequential mutations in one cell line.
C Latent period between initiation and death: ten years in males, twenty in females.

Another condition typical of old age is fracture of the neck of the

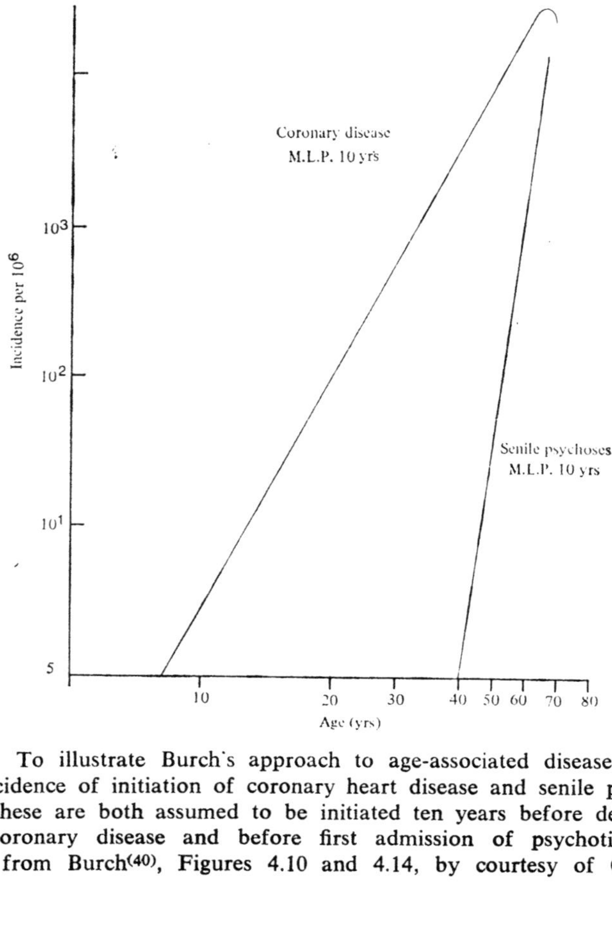

Figure 12 To illustrate Burch's approach to age-associated disease. The age-specific incidence of initiation of coronary heart disease and senile psychoses—in males these are both assumed to be initiated ten years before death in the case of coronary disease and before first admission of psychotic patients. (Redrawn from Burch[40], Figures 4.10 and 4.14, by courtesy of Oliver and Boyd.)

femur, the age-specific incidence of which gives a straight line with a slope of 7.0, i.e. it is accurately proportional to the 7th power of the age, and $r = 8$.

Burch's results are impressive to a non-mathematician and must indicate certain etiological regularities. As a biologist, however, I find some serious difficulties in his handling of the concepts of multiple somatic mutations that are essential in his equations. Mutations are, by definition, rare and informationally random. If we adhere to the usual convention of measuring any rate of mutation in terms of the probability of a specific type of mutation per cell generation, we automatically assume that mutation equals error at replication of a DNA segment. Earlier, reasons have been given for accepting the axiom that no mutation will result in an experimentally or clinically demonstrable change unless subsequent proliferation of the mutant cell, relative to unchanged cells, established a large enough mutant population for its new character to be recognized. In principle, it is only the *last* mutation of a series which demands a high proliferative advantage. If four sequential mutations are necessary to initiate the visible change, the first three need not necessarily induce a proliferative advantage at any of the mutational steps. The difficulty here is the very much higher mutation rate that would be necessary than if there were such proliferative advantages. This in fact has been raised as a major objection to the somatic mutation theory of ageing; the rate required is quite unacceptably high.

The basic contention in Burch's general theory is that multiple mutations must be accumulated until the necessary combination from which a clone of effectively autoaggressive cells can be built up, or, in the second type of equation, until n separate clones can develop simultaneously. If one adopts the most widely accepted view of the cellular dynamics of immunity—and in doing so sets aside Burch and Burwell's[(51)] elaborations of lymphocytic function—the susceptible population is the stem cell–lymphocyte–plasma cell series. It is an actively proliferating population throughout life, the end cells at least being highly expendable and rapidly replaced. One must assume that proliferation is going on in all 'compartments', from the stem cell onwards, with corresponding opportunities for selective proliferation of mutants.

Unfortunately extremely little is known, or perhaps can be known, of the process of immunocyte diversification by mutation or pseudomutation during the phases before the results of the changes are expressed. Burch may be justified in assuming that in this cell population somatic mutation occurs at a high enough rate for there to be no necessity for the first $(r - 1)$ mutations to have any significant proliferative advantage. With the rth mutation, the mutant, by hypothesis, is the fully developed autoaggressive cell which will be stimulated to active proliferation by the corresponding autoantigen. The time needed for the final proliferation to give a large enough clone to produce symptoms of disease is allowed for in Burch's graphs by adopting an appropriate latent period between initiation and manifestation of the index sign or symptom. The absence from his equations of any term, other than this one, concerned with proliferative advantage of the mutant is not a serious objection to the approach, provided it is recognized that relatively high rates of somatic mutation are called for. Where more than one kind of mutation is necessary in distinct cells in type (1) equations, there is considerably greater difficulty in giving a biological interpretation to the interaction of *n* distinct mutant lines from which disease is initiated. The existence of multiple antibodies, as in systemic lupus, may well be secondary results of a primary process involving T-cells, possibly a single clone only, possibly more than one. As will be discussed later, there is a growing opinion that both tolerance and its converse, autoimmune disease, are usually reflections of T-cell function. There are examples of pure B-cell tolerance and some autoimmune diseases where B-cells must be primarily concerned, but they are rare. Until much more is known of T-cell somatic genetics and immunological function, it will remain very difficult to give an adequate cellular interpretation of Burch's diagrams and deductions.

Burch's interpretation of all non-malignant age changes as manifestations of autoimmune processes also seems biologically extremely unlikely. It is almost inconceivable how any sequence of seven or eight mutations in a single line of immunocytes could dominate the etiology either of fracture of the neck of the femur or death from coronary disease. If we consider the increased vulnerability of bones to fracture as the simpler situation, it seems unnecessary to call on autoimmune processes at all. A simpler explanation is that the steep increase of incidence with age depends on the accumulation with age of a relatively large set of mutational impairments in the various tissues concerned. A considerable proportion doubtless depend on mutations accumulating in the cell lines most directly involved, i.e. the collagen-producing cells of bony tissue.

It may be wise for the present to keep an open mind on the possibility that most of the observed degenerative conditions of old age are autoimmune in type. It is just conceivable that there is a nearly universal development of 'aggressive' autoimmune clones of T-lymphocytes reactive against fibroblasts and causing the production of less and poorer quality collagen or against vascular endothelium with damage that initiates atherosclerosis and its secondary effects. Until there is definite experimental evidence of the existence of such cells, however, it is a possibility to be kept in the background.

There can be no question of the value of Burch's general approach to the analysis of the age-specific incidence of chronic human disease. Any advance toward understanding what happens during senescence will require continuing use and improvement of his methods of deducing the relevant parameters by stochastic analysis of epidemiological data. The implicit assumption of an autoimmune etiology for all degenerative conditions, however, imposes unnecesary limitation. The implications of Orgel error-catastrophe processes could certainly be put into stochastic-mathematical form and applied to relevant manifestations of ageing or age-associated disease, wherever it seemed likely to be useful. From the broader point of view it seems desirable to seek a combined mathematical–biological study of the whole range of observable results from somatic mutation. This would include mutant clone proliferation with its direct (neoplastic) and indirect (autoimmune) pathological results, and self-accelerating processes of sequential mutation leading to error catastrophe. In due course it may become possible to apply appropriate mathematical treatment to mutation in non-proliferating (post-mitotic) cells in the central nervous system and elsewhere. All four types of consequence seem to be concerned in ageing and will need quantitative interpretation in any comprehensive theory.

What worries many people about Burch's theories and their mathematical formulation is that they leave no place for environmental factors. I have written much about the vastly commoner tendency to look *only* for enviromental factors—viral, toxic, chemical, or physical—in diseases not easily understood, but I find I have a little of the same sort of prejudice against ascribing the etiology of any disease *wholly* to genetic and somatic genetic factors. I continue to try to occupy an intermediate position, but it is a good deal closer to Burch's than to that of the confirmed environmentalists. In fact, if a good deal of agnosticism is allowed on both sides, I believe that our points of view on ageing are compatible.

Curtis's somatic mutational theory

Curtis[52] has developed a somatic mutational approach to ageing which is less closely related to our central theme. He observed that chromosomal abnormalities in regenerating liver cells of mice increased steadily with age and regarded the changes as indicative of mutation, more likely multiple than single, taking place in non-proliferating cells. The method used to detect chromosomal changes was to cause partial necrosis of liver cells with carbon tetrachloride and examine the liver cell nuclei 72 hours later, when regeneration was at its peak. The proportion of nuclei showing distortion of mitotic pattern was assessed as a measure of the level to which somatic mutations has accumulated in the liver.

This technique was applied to a number of situations relevant to ageing, using mice for most experiments. When a short-lived strain, A, was compared with long-lived C57B1, the proportion of liver cells showing chromosomal aberrations rose more rapidly in the short-lived than the longer-lived strain; and more rapidly in mice than in dogs, which have a sixfold longer lifespan. There were, however, discrepancies. A very short-lived strain, C58, with a median lifespan of ten months and death almost always resulting from leukaemia, showed no increased chromosomal aberrations in liver cells. F1 hybrids of short-lived and long-lived mouse strains showed an intermediate incidence of chromosomal changes, but like most F1s they had a longer lifespan than either parent strain.

In addition to the strain differences in mice, Curtis's main findings were on the effect of X-irradiation known to produce a shortening of lifespan in mice in comparison with a toxic chemical agent which had no such effect. Sublethal treatment with X-rays was effective in increasing the characteristic liver cell abnormalities beyond those appropriate to chronological age. Nitrogen mustard has a well known damaging effect on DNA, but even at a dose that killed 50 per cent of the mice there was no effect on lifespan of the survivors and these showed only a normally rising level of chromosomal anomalies with age.

A comparison of the rate at which liver cell abnormalities developed spontaneously in the three species, mouse, guinea-pig, and beagle-dog, showed that the rate diminished, in that order, in parallel with the average lifespans of two, six and twelve years respectively.

A theoretical point of considerable interest is that there is very little normal turnover of liver cells in the mouse, so that the changes responsible for the observed abnormalities are presumably taking place in non-multiplying cells. There is, however, a high and probably variable metabolic activity of liver cells. The associated activities in the nucleus could on occasion call for repair of DNA and provide opportunity for error. The exact nature of the interference with chromosomal function, resulting in bridging and other distortions, is obscure, and it seems likely that for the time being the changes should be regarded as a special form of age-related change only indirectly related to what is evident in lymphocytes and fibroblasts. An important point made by Curtis, which emphasizes the difference between the chromosomal aberrations he was studying and at least some other types of mutation, concerned the persistence of results induced by irradiation. When mice were given a substantial dose of X- or neutron-irradiation, there were two demonstrable results of subsequent treatment with CCl_4. The regenerating cells showed mitotic abnormalities in a much higher proportion than normal mice of the same age, and if the mice were allowed to survive, a high proportion developed hepatomas. With increasing delay before testing the animals with CCl_4, the proportion of chromosomal anomalies steadily fell, and at nine months it was nearly down to normal level. The heightened proportion of hepatomas, however, remained about the same.

Curtis's general conclusion is that somatic mutation is the dominating factor in the process of ageing, and that most of the significant effects arise from mutation in cells which do not normally undergo clonal proliferation. He is impressed with the complexity of the situation and believes that virtually all the signs and symptoms of ageing represent the combined effects of multiple and sequential mutations. He has a general sympathy with Burch's approach and, like him, postulates that the rate of mutation does not increase with age.

This is probably an appropriate place to say something about a point made strongly by Curtis, that mutation is more important when it involves fixed cells with little or no normal turnover, such as those in the liver, rather than in those that undergo continual clonal proliferation, such as the lymphocytes and their precursors. The view is widely held that wherever there is a rapid turnover with active production of new cells and a correspondingly high rate of elimination and death, any mutant, being presumably in some way less efficient, will have an increased likelihood of being eliminated. One of the examples commonly cited is the extreme rarity of carcinoma of the small intestine, where the lining epithelial cells are constantly being renewed from the muscosal crypts and thrown off into the gut. Tumours of the red cell line, with its very rapid turnover, are equally rare. In both cases, however, it must be remembered that the mature functional cell has lost the capacity for mitosis. The conditions are different where epithelial layers exposed to the environment are continually regenerating lost cells and repairing traumatized areas. It is at the points where regeneration and repair to deal with chronic trauma are most active that carcinoma is most prone to arise, on exposed areas of skin, the cervix uteri, bronchial mucosa, and in the gastrointestinal tract toward the pyloric end of the stomach, and in large bowel and rectum. Here we are using the appearance of malignancy simply as an index of the extent of somatic mutation in the region. If diffuse somatic mutations of all sorts in proliferating cells represent an important part of the increasing functional ineffectiveness of the old, we should expect to see the same cell systems involved. To a large extent this is the case.

Among the cardinal features of ageing are thinning of the skin and loss of hair pigmentation; atrophy of the gastric mucosa is usual and often severe. One observation that constitutes a partial exception is the atrophy of connective tissue and collagen-producing cells. Sarcomas of subcutaneous tissue and bone are not common, perhaps because there is no special area exposed to additional irritation. The statistics of age incidence of bone cancer (i.e. sarcoma), however, show a perfectly typical age-associated curve, which could well be correlated with degeneration of collagen-producing cells through accumulating somatic mutations.

Life-shortening by X-irradiation

A large part of medical discussion on the part played by somatic mutation in ageing has centred on the life-shortening effect of relatively heavy X-irradiation of experimental animals. The topic has already been mentioned incidentally and it is convenient to include in this chapter some further notes on the effect of irradiation on lifespan.

As Walford points out[47], the significance of life-shortening by X-irradiation is hard to analyse. There is no doubt about the effect; a total dose of 5000 R, distributed over the whole life of the mouse, doubles the rate of ageing. When a single acute dose of 200–400 R is used, the life-shortening effect is most marked in one-day-old mice, and and in experiments reported by Lindhop and Rotblat[53, 54], mice at forty weeks showed the least effect, with seventy-two-week-old animals more sensitive. The incidence of diseases of ageing was not greatly modified apart from appearing earlier than in unirradiated mice. This held for malignant tumours as well as for degenerative conditions for all groups with one exception. This was a *decrease* in tumour incidence in mice given the highest dose (780 R) at thirty days of age. If, as the authors suggested, this was a therapeutic effect, it would indicate that in thirty-day-old mice potential cancer-producing cells are already in existence. This finding could be highly relevant in relation to the function of immunological surveillance discussed in Chapter 14.

A single dose of X-rays is more effective in shortening the lifespan than the same dose given over a prolonged period, which is the general rule for biological effects of radiation.

Not all the standard parameters of ageing are affected by irradiation.

Walford notes that in hamsters irradiated at three months of age there was no change from the controls in the proportion of soluble collagen or in the accumulation of pigment in the myocardium.

Whole body irradiation of mice with single X-ray doses of 200–600 R has a sharp effect on the thymus, with necrosis of cortical cells and atrophy of the whole organ. Similar results are seen with radiomimetic drugs, such as cyclophosphamide. Both types of agent are well known for their capacity to suppress immune responses.

For reasons previously discussed, any accelerated production of somatic mutations by X-irradiation cannot be recognized directly in the living animal though it can be shown to occur in cell cultures. The observed effect on lifespan is likely to be predominantly a result of damage to the thymus and T-immune system. One can be certain that many somatic mutations and other forms of nuclear damage result from large doses of irradiation, but these will only be recognized when proliferative (i.e. neoplastic) processes are induced.

CHAPTER 8

THE THYMUS IN RELATION TO AGEING

Increasing vulnerability to infection is one aspect of ageing which may well be responsible for the terminal breakdown in a majority of natural deaths. Enough direct evidence is available that various measurable functions of the immune system show progressive weakening and inefficiency with age. Presumably this must in some way be related to accumulating somatic mutational changes in lymphocytes and their derivates, perhaps particularly in T-immunocytes. At one stage I was inclined to look on the striking atrophy and eventual almost complete disappearance of the thymus as an index of the process by which T-cell immune function faded out. That may well be partially true, but for the present it is probably better to concentrate attention on the lymphocytes as a model system of clonally proliferating cells and try to understand the manifestations of cumulative somatic mutational changes in such a system.

Since Jacques Miller's first publication(55), in 1961, on the effect of removal of the thymus in new-born mice, there has been both a flood of investigations on the thymus and a growing unanimity about its importance in controlling one major segment of immune reactivity. At least one research group, Bede Morris and his colleagues at Canberra, is sceptical about the importance that most other immunologists ascribe to the thymus. Their experimental animal, the sheep, can tolerate the loss of its thymus half way through its foetal life with remarkable little effect on the lamb after birth. This is an important result, but the self-consistency of what is observed in mice and its apparent relevance to a variety of immune deficiency diseases in man is too impressive to allow us to discard the hypothesis because it does not seem to hold for the sheep.

The function of the thymus

The following account of the thymus is drawn from experimental work in mice and from clinical and pathological studies in man[56]. It is necessarily oversimplified and, where controversy still exists, the interpretation that fits most logically with the rest is accepted.

The most obvious feature of the thymus is its change in size and composition with age. Its size, relative to the rest of the body, is greatest around the time of birth—about a month before birth in man, a week or two after birth in the mouse. Its greatest absolute weight is reached in adolescence—around ten to twelve years in man. It thrinks rapidly at puberty and thereafter it dwindles steadily in size, the lymphoid tissue being progressively replaced by fat and fibrous tissue. After the age of fifty there is still a remnant of characteristic shape, but it has virtually no functional tissue.

The thymus at its prime in early childhood has a thick outer layer, the cortex of close-packed lymphocytes, often referred to as thymocytes, multiplying more rapidly than the cells in any other tissue of the body. The essential component of its atrophy with age is a reduction in the amount and number of the cortical lymphocytes, resulting in a progressive diminution in the number of new clones of thymus-dependent cells being set free into the circulation to reach the lymph nodes, spleen, and other peripheral accumulations of lymphoid cells.

For an interpretation of cellular changes, experimental work on mice must be used, but it seems almost certain that similar processes go on in man. Thymus-dependent lymphocytes (also referred to as T-immunocytes or just T-cells) can be distinguished in several ways from the B-lymphocytes, which, as described earlier, appear to differentiate in the bone marrow and are wholly responsible for producing free antibody. There is still some controversy on the matter, but I accept work at the Hall Institute by Marchalonis and others[57] as indicating that T-cells synthesize and carry on their surface antibody or antibody-like material to serve as a receptor specifically tuned to react with a corresponding antigen. They do not, however, liberate any significant quantity of antibody into the blood plasma or tissue fluids. The function of these thymus-dependent cells can be described fairly correctly as to seek out and destroy any cells which they can recognize as alien to the body.

Such alien cells may be parasites, but more often they are cells of the body rendered recognizably alien by a virus, by the attachment of antigens from microorganisms, or—and this is of special importance—by genetic abnormalities of the somatic cells. Experimentally, it is easy to expose the body to genetically abnormal cells by simply transplanting a piece of skin from an animal of the same species but unrelated to the recipient. As is well known, such a foreign graft is always rejected by a normal animal, and it is the T-cells which are mainly responsible. Miller's key experiment[55] was to remove the thymus surgically from new-born mice and when they were a few weeks old test them for capacity to reject skin grafts from mice of an unrelated strain. In contrast to the normal rejection by the control mice, the grafts remained healthy for long periods. Even rat skin could be successful transplanted. At a later stage (see page 161), mutant cells carrying new or altered antigens will need to be considered extensively in relation to various neoplastic conditions. Everything points to the T-cell system being an important protective agent against all such potentially pathogenic mutant cells.

One of the significant developments of immunology in the past five years has been the increasing importance that is being ascribed to T-cells. It has been accepted for some time that most antigens can only induce antibody formation as a result of a complex interaction involving specific activation of both T- and B-cells by antigen, and often requiring in addition the cooperation of macrophages. There is still controversy about the detail of these interactions but, whatever the final decision, the results as they stand have important applications to immune tolerance and the various manifestations of autoimmunity. Very few, perhaps none, of the potential antigens in the body belong to the limited class of antigens for which B-cells can be stimulated to produce antibody without benefit of T-cell cooperation. This means, or may mean, that B-cells of types which could react with potential antigens in the body may often be present but are inert in the absence of T-cells which could react with the self antigen in question. In other words, natural tolerance of body antigens may depend wholly on there being a strict censorship of T-cells in the thymus to eliminate or inhibit all that can react with accessible body antigens.

On this view, most autoimmune disease may be manifestation of somatic mutational change in T-cells only, and the production of autoantibodies a mere secondary effect not necessarily entailing parallel mutation in B-cells.

In the conventional area of defence against microorganisms, control of acute bacterial infections is mainly the responsibility of B-cells and the antibodies they produce, but most infections due to viruses, slow growing bacteria like the tubercle bacillus, and pathogenic fungi are dealt with predominantly by the T-cell system. In practice the efficiency of the T-cells is usually tested by the use of a small battery of 'skin tests'. A typical example is the Mantoux test, in which a dilute solution of a protein produced by the tubercle bacillus is injected into the skin. A positive reaction—a dark red, slightly swollen patch coming up 24–48 hours after the injection—means that the person has at some time been infected, usually harmlessly, with tuberculosis. Most people will also have been infected during childhood with several other common micro-organisms that give similar type skin reactions with the appropriate extracts. In all a positive means that (*a*) the person has been infected in the past by the corresponding organism and (*b*) his T-cells are functioning normally. When a paediatrician is concerned about a child who may have an immune deficiency disease, an important part of his investigation is to assess the patient's capacity to react to tests of this sort. Failure to react to those that would be expected to be positive points toward a deficiency of the thymus-dependent immune system.

Appropriate experiments show that there is a steady traffic of cells through the thymus. Stem cells arrive from the bone marrow, implant in the cortex, and proliferate. In the process they develop the surface receptors which can be thought of as antibody molecules built into the cell membrane and which allow contact with and 'recognition' of the corresponding antigen. At this stage they are called antigen-reactive cells and, most immunologists believe, are subject to an immediate 'censorship', by which any whose receptors react strongly enough with any of the hundreds of antigens present in the cells and fluids of the thymus are either switched to some other function or, more likely, killed and eliminated. Once the processes of differentiation and censorship are completed—they seem to take about twenty days in the mouse—T-cells that have survived the censorship pass into the blood and lodge eventually in spleen, lymph nodes, and other collections of lymphoid tissue.

Perhaps, as could be expected if the thymus is a 'rate-determining' organ, its growth seems to be largely autonomous. When a thymus from a young animal is transplanted to an old one, it grows as a young thymus, apparently unaffected by the age of its new host. Thymus from an old mouse shows no rejuvenation when grafted on to a young mouse.

An even more significant result is that one can transplant a dozen or more thymuses from young mice under the skin of an adult[58]. All will establish themselves and grow to about the normal size of a mouse thymus, unaffected by the fact that there is a wholly abnormal amount of thymic tissue in that mouse. No other transplanted organ is allowed such latitude.

The thymus as a biological clock

This outline of the immunological function of the thymus is very incomplete and a number of other aspects will be touched on in later pages. For the present it is intended simply to provide enough background to allow an understanding of those aspects of immunity that are associated with the general inefficiency of immune processes which is a common, and may be an invariable, feature of growing old. At one stage, largely influenced by Walford, I was prepared to think that the thymus and its dependent T-cells provide the most important of the 'biological clocks' which at the physiological level must determine when the appropriate lifespan for the species is being reached. It is almost certainly inappropriate to put the whole responsibility for lifespan on a single bodily system, and in later chapters much that will be said about age-associated disease is only indirectly related to changes in the immune system. Nevertheless it is easy to find persuasive reasons for the special importance of the thymus system, and, provided it is recognized that the general concept of intrinsic mutagenesis almost demands that all systems in the body must be involved in ageing, it may be worth while to pay special attention to the role of the thymus and develop the hypothesis that in one sense the thymus can play a major part in the timing of senescence.

Basically the hypothesis is that T-lymphocytes are necessary for health —to deal with many types of infection in cooperation with B-cells, to handle malignant and other changes in body cells, and in all probability to help counter autoimmune disease. If their number and quality are too far below standard, death will ensue. I have given the evidence that B-lymphocytes, and therefore presumably T-lymphocytes also, are subject to a limit on the number of cell generations they may undergo after once being specifically stimulated. Not everyone would agree that this has more than superficial analogies with Hayflick's phenomenon in cell cultures, but at least it indicates clearly that cell proliferation of certain clones cannot continue indefinitely. We can feel justified in developing the concept that, as long as clonally proliferating cells like lymphocytes remain non-malignant, there is some inbuilt limitation on the total number of cell generations they can produce.

What evidence there is suggests that between the entry of a stem cell into the thymus and the emergence of its descendants there are perhaps twenty cell generations, but that for a variety of reasons most of the cells produced die and their substance is worked over again in the thymus. Perhaps not more than a dozen cells emerge as differentiated T-cells for every stem cell that entered. In other words, the thymus uses up a lot of cell generations to provide only a small increase in numbers.

More than any other organ in the body the thymus is sensitive to stress. Any injury or illness that is severe enough to send a child or young adult to hospital results in the death of enormous numbers of lymphocytes in the cortex of the thymus and temporary atrophy of the organ. The thymus is very inaccessible in the top of the chest; it cannot be measured in the living individual. If an anatomist wants to know how large the human thymus is at each age, the only way he can obtain the information is by doing post-mortem examinations on victims of motor car accidents who have been killed immediately. A patient dying even twenty-four hours after the accident already shows gross changes in the thymus.

Most people recover from their accidents, their surgical operations, and their fevers, but each episode of stress means the loss of enormous numbers of thymus cells and an extra call on stem cells for restocking. With some rather complex mathematics we might be able to say that, starting with perhaps 100 stem cells that have differentiated far enough for them to be predestined to become T-lymphocytes, they can produce at most only a certain number of descendants. If each of those 100 cells on the average produces a clone that can continue for fifty generations, before it reaches its Hayflick limit all the cells of all generations in the clone would amount to 2×10^{15} if none failed to divide successfully. In fact there would be losses at every stage and the total would be far less. This sort of approach, however, would at least allow us to say that the thymus and the cells dependent on it are, as it were, allotted a 'quota' of potential descendant cells. A stressful early life with many illnesses will make exceptional demands on the quota and it will be exhausted abnormally early. One might expect that average age at death is related to the intensity of stress in early life, and there are figures to bear this out. It does not *prove* that premature exhaustion of the thymus helps toward early death, but it is consistent with the suggestion.

In trying to understand the possible role of exhaustion of thymic function in producing the immunological concomitants of age it is necessary to keep three distinct processes clearly in mind:

1. The characteristic time sequence of changes in the thymus of the normal individual is clearly keyed to the evolutionary needs of the immune system. In all probability their genetic control is dependent mainly on hormonal factors. Pituitary function is necessary for thymic development and the sharp reduction in the size of the thymus at puberty is largely a result of hormonal activity from the gonads. The other two processes are superimposed on this primary physiological pattern.
2. The influence of infection and other systemic stresses on the thymus, with their massive destruction of thymocytes, is quite unrelated to any intrusion of error into the process of cellular proliferation. It is merely a characteristic normal reaction of a proportion of lymphocytes to a heightened level of corticosteroids in circulation.
3. Limits to the proliferation of individual clones of the type demonstrated by Williamson and Askonas is only likely to be important after adolescene and to become critical only towards the end of life. Nevertheless it represents a direct continuation of the process of using up our hypothetical quota of cell generations.

The main weakness of any hypothesis that the thymus plays a major role in determining the time at which ageing becomes evident is the difficulty of devising any type of experiment that can be accepted as providing proof or disproof of the hypothesis. The obvious approach was to remove the thymus surgically in a young animal and see what effect this has on growth, resistance to disease, and longevity. Such experiments in dogs, rabbits and mice showed no obvious effect on the health of the animal and no one seems to have felt it worth while to see whether they had any influence on lifespan. Almost certainly the basic reason for this absence of effect is that most of the function of the thymus is carried out before birth or very soon afterwards. When an animal like a mouse, which is born in a relatively undeveloped state, has its thymus removed immediately after birth, the story is different. The loss of capacity to reject foreign skin grafts by such neonatally thymectomized mice has already been described. Such animals usually die around three months of age, but not from some acceleration of normal ageing. If mice born from mothers that have been raised in the absence of all bacteria are thymectomized at birth and themselves raised under germ-free conditions, they live much longer. Essentially, the early death is due to inability to handle bacteria and their toxins; whether there is any reduction in lifespan apart from this has not been established.

Although it is only indirectly relevant, recent work indicates that germ-free mice have a *shorter* lifespan than comparable conventionally reared animals[59]. Walford suggests that this could be related to the need for some degree of antigenic stimulation if the immune system is to mature normally.

Very little work has been done on the effect of thymectomy *after* the neonatal period on the lifespan of mice, but the only report I have found[60] showed that they died significantly earlier than sham-operated controls. Deaths were distributed in such a fashion as to suggest that the main deficiency was inadequacy in dealing with accidental infections rather than any more systematic process.

Genetic forms of thymic deficiency in mice

The other classical approach to organ function is to observe the effect of congenital failure of its development. The physiological importance of the thymus is so great that the only possibility of obtaining animals to work with is to find a double recessive condition in mice associated with complete or partial lack of a thymus and to maintain a heterozygous breeding stock. Two such strains are known: 'Nude' and Snell–Bagg, animals of the first strain in which the homozygotes *nu*/*nu* are hairless, possess no thymus (though a small nodule of what might be thymic epithelium has been described), and show none of the classical activities of T-immunocytes. They will readily accept foreign grafts of skin or tumours, including human tumours. They are prone to infection and die between three and seven months of age. However, Pantelouris[61] finds that if young *nu*/*nu* mice are given a thymus graft from compatible heterozygotes *nu*/+, they grow and show increased resistance to infection. Unlike the standard 'nude', they are fertile, and mating of treated male and female has produced uniform *nu*/*nu* offspring.

The most impressive experimental evidence in favour of the importance of the thymus in ageing comes from the work of Swiss investigators, Fabris, Pierpaoli and Sorkin[62], on the Snell–Bagg strain. Like the nude strain, Snell–Bagg mice are the homozygous manifestation of a recessive gene. The stock must similarly be maintained in the heterozygous form in which each parent has one dose of the faulty gene. One fourth of their offspring will be Snell–Bagg mice and these show all the signs of accelerated ageing. The mice die at an age of three months, with wrinkled skin, and marked thinning and greying of the hair. There are two ways of correcting the process. One is by injection of growth hormone and thyroxine; the second is by injecting lymph node cells from normal heterozygotes of the same strain. The crucial experiment is that when the thymus is removed from the prematurely ageing homozygote, subsequent administration of growth hormone and thyroxine is *not* effective in normalizing the animal. The most direct interpretation of the results is that the function of the thymus depends on normal production of growth hormone and thyrotrophic hormone by the pituitary. If this fails, the thymus cannot provide the conditions that allow the differentiation and liberation of the T-cells. This failure of the pituitary is the essential weakness of the Snell–Bagg mice. There may be harmful effects on other organs, but the effectiveness of an injection of lymphocytes shows that the thymus effect is the most important. In the double recessive Snell–Bagg mice the thymus can neither function itself nor endow thymus-like qualities on other lymphoid tissues, and in the absence of T-cells the ageing process is preternaturally rapid. If the effect is to be remedied by hormone administration, T-cells are required and a thymus must be present to produce them. On the other hand, when T-cells from a heterozygous animal with normal hormones are injected directly, the abnormal ageing is equally well counteracted.

That interpretation will probably prove to be unduly simplified when more extensive studies of the Snell–Bagg mice are made. The double recessive syndrome, with early death, as seen in these two mouse strains, may have only a superficial resemblance to natural ageing. At the present time, however, it is the best experimental model that has been provided. As so often happens in physiology, experiments of nature in which there is genetic excision of an organ's function can often be more illuminating than the results of surgical removal.

Pituitary influences

Immunologists have rarely paid much attention to the effect of endocrinological and metabolic factors on the functioning of the immune system. Yet it is obvious that if the interpretation of experiments with the Snell-Bagg mice is correct, the pituitary gland at least plays an important role in immunity. With a little thought on such relationships it becomes obvious that any formulation of theories dealing with ageing, immunity, growth or repair must be made with the full understanding that they represent only limited aspects of the organism as a whole. For growth, repair, and the immune responses, as for all other bodily functions, the circulating blood must maintain a proper internal environment for all tissues. This means, among many other things, that all the needed hormones must be available at the right times and at the right levels of concentration in the blood.

At one time there was a fashion to ascribe many of the manifestations of ageing to the disappearance of the sex hormones. There was a glorious age of scientific quackery in the 1890s when rejuvenation of the elderly rich was offered by the implantation of 'monkey glands'. That phase soon passed, but, ever since, there has been serious interest in hormonal aspects of ageing, with much of the attention focused on the pituitary.

There are two sets of observations which at first sight seem to offer no relationship whatever to an immunological theory of ageing. Both are unequivocal and have been frequently confirmed. In looking for corerlations between lifespan and the size and anatomical structure of different species of mammal, the only 'good' correlation that has been established is with the index of cephalization, i.e. a relationship of size of brain to body weight. Sacher[63] developed the formula $\log x = 0.6 \log z - 0.23 \log y + 0.99$, where x is the lifespan in years, y body weight, and z brain weight, both in grams. Man is probably the longest-lived mammal, and, among dogs, the relatively large-brained Pekinese lives twenty years to the St. Bernard's twelve to fourteen.

The second is the well known effect of restricted diet due to McCay[64]. Young rats were given, from the time of weaning, a qualitatively adequate diet, but with a calorie deficiency sufficient to slow their growth to almost zero. This diet could be continued for more than two years, and if the rats were then given normal diet, they developed rapidly and remained in good health for up to four years, which is more than a year beyond the normal span. It was notable that in such animals chronic pulmonary disease and tumours were much less prevalent than in normally raised animals.

Obviously both sets of observations must be fitted into any adequate interpretation of ageing. My own impression is that in both instances pituitary activity involving growth hormone is involved. This had been suggested long ago for the nutritional experiments by Samuels[65], who referred to the effect as a dietary hypophysectomy. Its application to the brain/body size relationship to lifespan is merely based on the predominant effect of growth hormone on the bones and other peripheral structures and not on the brain. One of the early experiments of H. M.

Evans on growth hormone[66] gave the rather striking result that rats hypophysectomized at six days after birth died of cerebral compression. The brain grew normally, but not the cranial skeleton. Administration of growth hormone to these animals without pituitaries allowed approximately normal growth. The conection between somatotrophic hormone and the immune system must be via the thymus if the Snell–Bagg mice experiments are valid and applicable in principle to other species. It would be analogous to what happens in other organs of internal secretion for the pituitary to control the synthesis and secretion of thymosin or any other local hormone liberated by the epithelial cells of the thymus. Such local hormones are generally accepted as playing a part in the production of immunocytes in the thymus and without them the thymus would be expected to remain permanently atrophic.

Amongst other possibilities, part of the increased lifespan of initially undernourished rats might conceivably be based on a markedly slowed turnover of stem cells in the thymus as a result of a chronic partial deficiency of pituitary hormones. This would allow the accumulation of a better balanced repertoire of immune patterns for mature life with better control as reported of chronic pulmonary infection and malignant tumours. There are clearly some interesting investigations of thymic physiology to be undertaken in these rats in relation both to dietary studies and to the result of surgical removal of the pituitary.

Another feature requiring brief discussion is the nature of puberty. In man this sets in about the age of twelve, and in adition to the development of secondary sexual characters it is associated with a sharp increase in growth rate. From our point of view it is equally important that about this time the thymus begins to decrease in size, as do the tonsils and perhaps other peripheral lymphoid accumulations. These puberal changes are largely related to steroid hormones from the gonads. Dougherty[67] has reviewed the reports on the action of testostenone and related substances on the mouse thymus. Injection of any of them causes a sharp reduction in the size of the thymus, presumably due to loss of cortical cells. This atrophy is a direct effect of testosterone, not something mediated through the adrenals. Puberty seems to mark the end of the period during which the child is, as it were, expected to develop its working repertoire of immunities. The stock of memory cells is adequate and the process of generating new immune patterns has become less urgent. The background of security against infection is there, on which hormonal and other aspects of maturity can develop.

CHAPTER 9

OTHER IMMUNOLOGICAL ASPECTS IN AGEING

The influence of immune factors in relation to ageing is important, perhaps pre-eminently important. An immunologist can well be excused for taking it as the central theme of his picture of ageing, and, as long as we remember that there are many ways of dying of old age for other reasons than the failure of defences against invading microorganisms or body cells rendered alien by malignant change, it is important to press the immunological approach as far as it will go. At this stage, therefore, a more specific account can be attempted of the main ways by which the postulated fading out of immune effectiveness is reflected in ageing. Four chief divisions can be recognized. The first concerns the extent and manifestations of falling antibody levels and eroded T-cell responses; the second deals with the manifestations of autoimmune disease and autoimmune processes generally in relation to age; the third sector deals with amyloid disease and the fourth with immune surveillance. This last will need to be deferred until the question of the relationship of the specific age-incidence of cancer with other aspects of the ageing process has been discussed in Chapters 11 and 12.

Age changes in effectiveness of the immune system

Most studies of changes in immunological efficiency with age have, for obvious reasons, been made in the most short-lived of the common laboratory animals, the domestic mouse. The capacity of mouse immunocytes to produce antibody against sheep red cells rises to a maximal level at about ten weeks of age and persists as a plateau to about forty weeks. Thereafter it falls progressively as the mouse ages[(68)]. Capacity to produce haemolytic antibody against sheep red cells is the most widely used test for antibody production in the mouse, but it must be recognized that for this antigen it is not simply a matter of stimulating B-immunocytes of appropriate pattern to multiply and synthesize antibody. The B-cells do actually produce the antibody, but both phagocytic cells (macrophages) and T-immunocytes must cooperate with antigen before an antibody-producing clone of B-cells can develop. The thymus therefore plays a part in the phenomena. An interesting experiment, due to Metclaf[(69)], involved surgical removal of the thymus in a largish group of young mice about two weeks old. These were tested, along with normal mice, for their response to the standard sheep red cell antigen. Tested in the first few months, there was no difference between the thymectomized animals and normal mice, but in another group, which were left untreated for eighteen months, the normal mice responded well but no antibody was produced by the thymectomized ones. The explanation almost certainly is that only while a thymus is present do 'new' lines of immunocytes keep on appearing. Old lines liberated into the circulation may persist for a long time, but in the absence of antigenic stimulation eventually become extinct, not necessarily by reaching a Hayflick limit, but from the various accidental hazards to which lymphocytes succumb.

The inability of old people to respond to new antigens, anthough they will give a typical active response to any that they had encountered earlier in life, is probably an example of the same phenomenon. A man of seventy has lost his thymus by effluxion of time just as effectively as if it had been surgically removed. Mackay's group in Melbourne studied the development and decline with age of antibody against flagellin from a Salmonella. The results[(70)] showed a peak between twenty and thirty, followed by a slow diminution with age. A specific stimulating injection of the antigen, however, gave as good a response in the old as in young adults. Many factors are involved in determining whether a man dies or recovers from infectious disease, but the effectiveness of the immune response must play an important part. When a community encounters a disease it has never previously met in epidemic form, the disease is most severe in the old. A graph of the mortality of patients against age shows almost regularly a smooth upward slope. The same heavy impact on the old is also seen in less exotic infections. Influenza is an excellent example. Many old people carry evidence of past experiences of influenza viruses in their blood streams and escape infection. In those with inadequate immunity to prevent or abort infection, a high mortality is likely.

Cell-mediated immunity, for which the T-immune system is responsible, shows a somewhat similar behaviour with age. In this field, however, there is very little experimental work with animals on record. A hint that the expected reduction in effectiveness occurs with age in guinea-pigs is given by Chase[(71)] in discussing the persistence of tolerance to skin-sensitizing chemicals. Standard tests indicated that the animals remained tolerant, i.e. non-reactive, indefinitely. The significance of that persistence was, however, rendered uncertain because old guinea-pigs frequently fail to become sensitized by procedures regularly effective on the young guinea-pigs routinely used in such experiments.

Much more extensive information is available at the clinical level. Old people not suffering from malignant disease show only a minor reduction, best seen in the very old, in their ability to become sensitized to standard antigens or skin-reactive chemicals. During the course of life most people encounter and overcome a variety of infections which can leave them sensitized to the corresponding antigen. Part of any comprehensive immunological study in hospital makes use of tests for skin sensitization with a battery of six or eight antigens of this type. Examples are those that indicate sensitization by the organisms responsible for tuberculosis, infantile thrush (*Candida*), mumps, and streptococcal infections. Most adults in an average hospital population will be sensitive to several of these. In an Australian hospital, systematic tests over a range of ages showed that fewer tests were positive in old age[(72)]. Of forty-five persons over eighty, only seventeen reacted positively to two or more antigens of the five which were used. From twenty to seventy-nine, there was only a slight diminution with age in the number of antigens giving positive reactions, the average falling from 3.8/5 to 2.9/5 in the group aged seventy to seventy-nine. In patients with clinically evident cancer, and especially in those with Hodgkin's disease, cell-mediated immunity of this type is strikingly less active than in people of the same age without cancer. It is still not clear whether lack of cell-mediated immunity favours the development of cancer or whether cancer as such depresses the activity of T-immune system.

Since the discovery of the first immuno-deficiency disease in 1956, about ten different types of deficiency capable of producing severe disease have been described[(73)]. They are all rare, but minor anomalies of all sorts are much more frequent. It is consistent with general biological experience and very much in line with the general tenor of this discussion of ageing to find an immense variety of minor immunological anomalies. Anyone who has ever tested the efficacy of some immunizing procedure on a large group of people by examining their subsequent antibody level will be aware of the wide scatter of results. Almost always a few will give no response. For fairly obvious reasons immunization with chemically pure antigens sharpens the differences amongst individuals. The important genetic differences between pure-line strains of guinea-pigs in their capacity to respond or not to respond by antibody production require rather simple synthetic antigens if they are to be clearly demonstrated.

Autoimmune disease

Autoimmune disease is by no means confined to old age, but there are several forms, such as rheumatoid arthritis, which are strongly age-related. One senses, too, a growing feeling that many, perhaps most, of the chronic degenerations and disabilities of the old have an autoimmune component. Another general impression, by no means properly validated, is that most of the autoimmune troubles of old age are, as it were, incidental results of the general inefficiency of immune mechanisms rather than specific responses to individual circumstances. At the present time it is impossible to present a comprehensive account of autoimmune disease in other than clinical and observational terms. Most immunologists are legitimately wary of general statements on the nature of intrinsic tolerance to body antigens and the various experimental types of immune unresponsiveness, and even more so in regard to the autoimmune phenomena which presumably follow from a breakdown of intrinsic tolerance. Nevertheless autoimmunity is obviously important in relation to ageing, and some attempt must be made to enumerate the main factors that seem to be concerned in autoimmune manifestations, particularly insofar as they are relevant to ageing.

1. It is a necessary condition of health that cells and tissues of the body should not be subject to the damaging attack by immunocytes and antibodies that is seen when foreign tissue is implanted. This does not necessarily mean that no reaction can occur with circulating substances normally in the blood nor with antigens accessible on the surface of body cells. It does demand that in one way or another the interaction has no pathological consequences.

2. On any currently acceptable view of the origin of specific immune

(antibody) pattern it is inevitable that immunocytes will emerge with receptors that are potentially reactive with this or that body antigen, and in one way or another they must be rendered inactive.

3. The nature of the immune tolerance that a healthy animal shows to its own components is highly controversial. I am still disposed to favour the simplest explanation that in general an animal is immunologically tolerant because there are no immunocytes in circulation that carry receptors whose immune patterns react with sufficient affinity on the accessible antigens to provoke clonal proliferation. Any current restatement of that position must make as clear a differentiation as can be justified of the parts played by T- and B-cells in tolerance. Probably present day majority opinion would centre tolerance on T-cells. In the absence of T-cell cooperation or some equivalent effect involving similar local concentration of the T-cell product, a normal B-cell, potentially reactive with body substance S, will remain inert in the presence of S. Its failure to proliferate or secrete antibody is a normal character, only to be overcome by an additional stimulus probably represented by a local concentration of an appropriate lymphokine.

Tolerance as a function of T-cells is a relatively new concept and may well have to be qualified in the future. It is, however, in line with the view, now coming back into popularity, that a major function of the thymus is as a censor for T-cells that have emerged with reactivity for self patterns. In the simplest form this censorship is envisaged as operating to ensure that as soon as a newly differentiated immunocyte with a pattern reactive with a body antigen emerges it is either killed or, what is operationally equivalent, inhibited from multiplying, by its first contact with the antigen.

4. When an autoimmune condition is gross enough to cause clinical disease, any form of the 'forbidden clone' hypothesis would require initiation of the condition by a somatic mutant immunocyte whose deviation from normal will differ according to whether it is a T-cell or a B-cell.

The aberrant T-cell is protected by the mutant character against inhibition or destruction by its first contact with the corresponding self antigen, normally in the thymus.

The pathogenic B clones found in most autoimmune haemolytic anaemias differ in being intrinsically susceptible to proliferate on contact with the corresponding self antigen, either in the absence of local lymphokine stimulation or requiring a lower intensity of lymphokine stimulation than normal.

In either case the clone has developed because the initiating cell and its descendants are genetically different from normal, presumably on account of a somatic mutation or a sequence of mutations which may include one or more of germ line origin. It is a 'forbidden clone' as a result.

5. Autoimmune disease requires the presence of the autoantigen in an accessible form and at a concentration which is effective in stimulating the pathogenic clone or clones to continue their proliferation.

6. All interactions between antigen and antibody or antibody-type receptor are non-covalent unions which may have any of a wide range of affinity levels. This holds both for normal immune responses and for autoimmune reactions. All antigen–antibody unions are initially reversible and modifiable by many circumstances. As a result, almost all generalizations in immunology are of a soft-edged quality; it is a 'very good' experiment that gives 90 per cent of the expected result. Most of the difficulties of understanding that arise at almost every step in work with autoimmune disease seem to derive from this soft-edged quality, plus the multiplicity of *types* of interaction that may come into play. One component of tolerance, for instance, may depend on antibody being present in sufficient amount to prevent antigen from stimulating T-immunocytes to destructive activity. Various lines of evidence suggest that there are several possible mechanisms that may interact to produce a 'fail-safe' situation which can minimize the damage associated with the escape of a forbidden clone from control.

Elaboration of most of these points can be found in recent discussion[30].

The type of cellular damage responsible for the signs and symptoms of autoimmune disease varies widely, but certain forms can be enumerated:

(i) The formation of circulating antigen-antibody complexes which may produce characteristic lesions in the kidney and sometimes in other tissues such as the joints. Most such antigen-antibody complexes are soluble in the presence of excess antigen, and if the autoantigen is a soluble protein present in the plasma, as is often the case, this will hold for the circulating blood. When passing into the tissues, e.g. the basement membrane of the kidney glomerulus, they are liable to be held and with the attachment of complement components produce local damage.

(ii) Antibody may act against cell surface receptors of a target organ mimicking hormonal stimulation. The only well established example[74] is the action of the autoantibodies 'LATS' and 'LATS-protector' in inducing thyrotoxicosis (exophthalmic goitre); there may be more.

(iii) Autoantibody may sensitize circulating red cells or platelets for removal in the spleen and elsewhere. This certainly occurs in autoimmune haemolytic anaemia, but there are many conditions in which red cells, to which antibody is attached as shown by a positive Coombs test, do not suffer rapid removal.

(iv) For obvious reasons, experimental and clinical studies of autoimmune disease have been much more directed towards antibodies than towards cell-mediated immunity and the other functions of T-cells, which, as indicated, may be specially important in the initiation of autoimmune disease. There is a special need for the development of methods for the recognition of monoclonal populations of T-cells with appropriate autoimmune specificity. What work has been done points to the likelihood that T-cells may be largely responsible for tissue damage, whereas much of the autoantibody recorded may be only significant in its capacity to protect potentially cytotoxic T-cells from activation by antigen.

The part played by autoimmune disease in ageing is still controversial. Burch's approach[(40)] has already been discussed in Chapter 7. He regards virtually all the degenerative processes of old age, including greying of hair and loss of teeth, and all the age-related diseases except cancer as showing the characteristic age-specific incidence of autoimmune processes. Such a conclusion may depend too much on a subtle mathematical analysis of biological processes that are not appropriate for such treatment. Most writers on the subject would doubt the universal role of autoimmunity but accept the close relationship of a number of autoimmune conditions with ageing. Of the well established diseases, rheumatoid arthritis increases its incidence with age in a fashion that suggests that about 50 per cent of individuals of both sexes are potentially susceptible, but the rate at which it becomes manifest is about twice as fast in women as in men.

Another important set of findings concerns the increasing incidence of autoantibodies with age (Figure 13). This is taken from an Australian investigation (of which I have some first-hand knowledge) dealing with more than 90 per cent of the population of a country town in Western Australia. The mass health survey is described by Cullen[(75)] and the immunological findings by Hooper *et al*[(76)]. A general review of these and related findings by Mackay has recently been published[(77)]. As

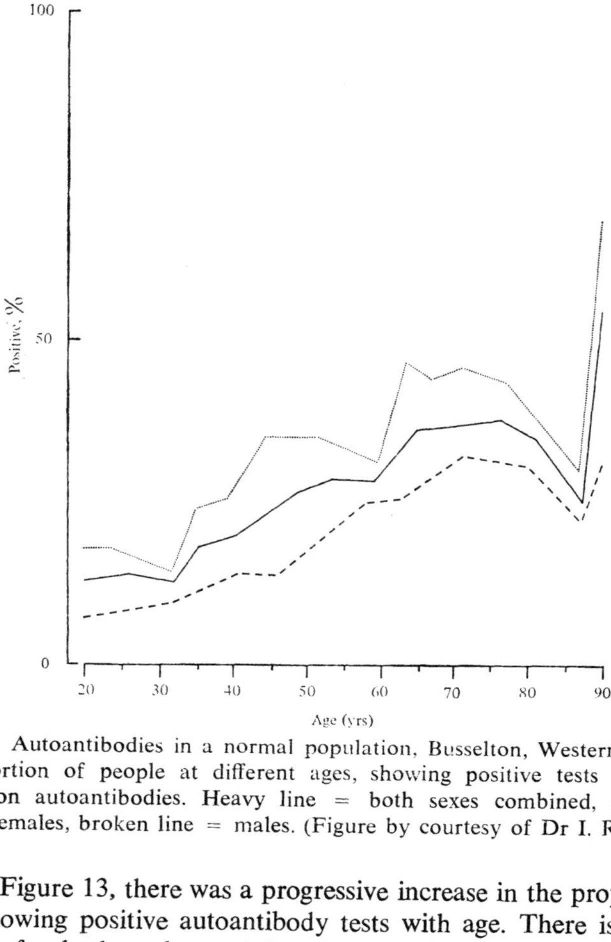

Figure 13 Autoantibodies in a normal population, Busselton, Western Australia. The proportion of people at different ages, showing positive tests for any of the common autoantibodies. Heavy line = both sexes combined, dotted line above = females, broken line = males. (Figure by courtesy of Dr I. R. Mackay.)

shown in Figure 13, there was a progressive increase in the proportion of people showing positive autoantibody tests with age. There is a dip in the curve for both males and females about the age of seventy-five, which could be an artifact. Reasons for accepting it as real can be found in three circumstances: (*a*) the ninety-seven Busselton subjects who died after the 1969 survey had more autoantibodies than a comparable age and sex matched sample from the same population that had survived; (*b*) a similar dip was seen in a study of immunoglobulin levels—which also rise with age—by Acheson and Jessop[78]; (*c*) Kipshidze[79] found a similar low level of gammaglobulin in the seventy to seventy-nine age group compared with the age groups on either side. One suggestion is that there are two populations concerned, one with the standard lifespan of sixty-five to seventy, the other of eighty to eighty-five, and that in both a rise in the proportion with autoantibodies is indicative of a major process leading to death. If these findings are confirmed, the phenomenon may become one of the main supports for ascribing much importance to autoimmunity in the final operative stage of ageing.

In experimental work perhaps the most striking influence of autoimmune disease as a life-shortening condition is the behaviour of the F1 hybrid mice (NZB × NZW) which develop several manifestations of autoimmune disease and die with regularity at less than 400 days of age, always from renal failure. Life can be greatly prolonged by treatment of the mice with cyclophsphamide[80]. Some strains of 'normal' mice show an increasing incidence of autoantibodies (specifically anti-nuclear factor) with age. This was found for the stock 'Hall Institute' strain by Norins and Holmes[81].

At several points already there have been hints that the general rundown of the immune system with age may in itself be responsible for some of the increased frequency of autoimmune disease in old age. It will be more convenient to discuss this at a later stage in relation to the lymphoreticular malignancies and related conditions (Chapter 15), but brief mention should be made here of Jerne's recent concept of the whole immune mechanism as an eigen system with a very large number of controlling interactions amongst cells, antibodies and antigens. The overall result, as everywhere in the internal environment, is to maintain homeostasis at optimal levels for bodily function. Diffuse accumulation of error-prone genetic mechanisms and inefficient enzymes in the cells of the system will progressively destroy that capacity for homeostasis. Susceptibility to death from infection to autoimmune disease and to amyloid deposition might all be ascribed in general terms to such failure of immune homeostasis. One probable example from experimental work may, however, be mentioned. Sutherland *et al.*[82] found that in rabbits from which thymus and appendix had been removed at birth, and which had subsequently been X-irradiated, positive Coombs tests and other manifestations of autoimmunity were common in later life. Here we have another association of autoimmune disease with partial crippling of the immune system.

Amyloid disease and ageing

The occurrence of amyloid degeneration of liver, kidney and spleen at autopsy of persons dying of tuberculosis or chronic sepsis has been known for centuries. It was thought to resemble starch (hence the name amyloid) and was identified in sections as an amorphous degenerate material, staining specifically with the dye, Congo red. Only in the last few years has there been any useful elucidation of the nature of the amyloid material or of the pathogenesis of its deposition. Now everything points to amyloid deposition being an immunological process occurring in an immune system under stress and inadequately controlled. It is also becoming increasingly evident that deposition of amyloid is almost a constant feature of ageing in man and probably most domesticated or experimentally used mammals. According to Walford[(47)], amyloidosis of at least mild degree is found post mortem in the great majority of people dying after their eightieth year. 'Senile plaques' of uncertain origin are found in the brain in about 50 per cent of old people. They appear to contain amyloid and are usually associated with typical amyloid deposition elsewhere in the brain and in other parts of the body. The pancreatic islets of Langerhans appear to be particularly commonly involved.

There has been little study of amyloid disease in relation to the normal ageing of laboratory animals. It is regularly seen in the hamster, the proportion of animals involved rising to 50 per cent at around two years of age. Amyloid is said to be common in ageing cattle, dogs and baboons, and may well be one of the commonest of the age-associated diseases of mammals.

There is a wide range of conditions associated with amyloid disease, and a brief list of the more important ones will indicate some of the difficulties of interpreting its pathogenesis.

In man: Chronic sepsis or tuberculosis, the classical associates, are now of course rarely seen; myelomatosis and other monoclonal gammopathies; familial Mediterranean fever and some other familial conditions; rheumatoid arthritis; Hodgkin's disease and other chronic neoplastic conditions; congenital agammaglobulinaemia. There are cases of 'spontaneous' amyloidosis in which no cause is apparent; this is a relatively common situation in New Guinean indigenes.

In other mammals: Injection of relatively large amounts of casein is the standard experimental procedure, but the condition may be found in other types of hyperimmunization; many horses used for commercial immunization develop amyloid.

The paradoxical feature immediately evident is that amyloid is produced in conditions associated with high immune activity and much immunoglobulin production, but also in a number of conditions where immune capacity is depressed: immunodeficiency diseases, Hodgkin's and other neoplastic diseases, and old age. This in itself suggests that an understanding of amyloidosis, on the one hand, and of the mechanism of ageing, on the other, would be mutually helpful.

In regard to the nature of amyloid it is now accepted[83] that the characteristic material is in the form of protein fibrils, which in tissues may be either intracellular or extracellular, associated with considerable amounts of degenerate cellular material and often with recognizable plasma cells and lymphocytes. Two distinct proteins have been obtained from amyloid fibrils, referred to by Hobbs[84] and others as A and B. The latter is at present the better understood. This B amyloid protein is of variable molecular weight (5000–31 000) and has been established as fragments of κ or λ light chains modified in some way which renders them highly resistant to proteolytic enyzmes. Almost identical material has been produced *in vitro* by the action of proteolytic enzymes on Bence-Jones protein. Clearly, one important type of amyloid degeneration is associated with the deposition of immunoglobulin. A second component, also a protein (A), has a molecular weight of 7000–8000 with no structural resemblance to immunoglobulin. Both A and B are likely to be found in all types of amyloid, but, characteristically, B is conspicuous mainly in conditions with monoclonal immunoglobulins circulating in the blood while A protein is more characteristic of amyloid, resulting from chronic sepsis, familial Mediterranean fever, and rheumatoid arthritis. The A protein can be shown to have specific antigenicity, and fluorescent antibody prepared against it is as satisfactory as Congo red for the histological identification of amyloid. From its distribution, Hobbs considers that amyloid A must, like amyloid B, be derived from some product of the immune system circulating in the blood, but so far nothing has been identified.

The interpretation of the pathogenesis of amyloid due to Cathcart *et al.*[85] seems likely to be the most relevant to conditions associated with ageing. It must necessarily be incomplete, but it will serve as a basis for discussion. They suggest that amyloidosis results from the death and subsequent autolysis of specific immunocytes—either plasma cells or T-cells.

The experimental basis for the hypothesis depends on the use of the MIF test for functional activity of T-cells stimulated by antigen. Lymphocytes from a sensitized animal, usually a guinea-pig, when mixed with antigen, release an agent, migration inhibitory factor (MIF), which prevents the normally active migration of macrophages in cell culture.

In guinea-pigs repeatedly injected with casein, a positive MIF reaction with casein is observed two weeks after the first injection, indicating sensitization and the presence of significant numbers of T-cells specific for casein. By four weeks the MIF reaction becomes negative and remains so for as long as the casein injections continue. This desensitization is specific to the casein, since simultaneous sensitization to some other antigen persists even when amyloidosis is well developed. The suggestion by Cathcart *et al.* is that all T-cells reactive with casein have in some way been eliminated.

The process by which amyloid is deposited in these guinea-pigs is obviously a complex one. If, as everything seems to suggest, amyloid is the partially autolysed and modified debris of dead immunocytes and their immunoglobulins, we have to find some reason for the localization of the process of cell death and autolysis. One can hardly avoid postulating a continuous production of T- and B-cells reactive with casein in some of the lymphoid tissues of the body and their simultaneous death and necrosis in the preferred sites of amyloid deposition. One can picture a local situation, perhaps initiated by the deposition of antigen–antibody complexes, where any sensitized T-cells would be stimulated by the abundant casein antigen to liberate lymphokines which could damage, often lethally, any adjacent lymphocytes, T or B, as well as themselves. Further deposition of casein as antigen–antibody complexes would occur at these sites and an autocatalytic process set in motion which would soon eliminate all reactive T-cells. An amyloid enhancing factor has been described by Janigan and Druet[86] whose chemical nature is uncertain but which could probably be accepted as a lymphokine. It might well mediate the local autocatalytic process that has been postulated.

To flood the circulation of a mouse or guinea-pig with casein is at best only a distant analogy to the long continued septic processes that produced classical amyloid disease in the days before antibiotics. The high frequency of amyloid in the old is nowadays not dependent on chronic infection but is in some way related to the high immunoglobulin level in the blood, which is one of the characteristic changes of old age. Most of this hyperglobulinaemia is probably associated with autoimmune processes.

One of the comon associations of amyloid disease is with multiple myelomatosis, with its characteristic high level of monoclonal immunoglobulin in the blood. Like the whole group of monoclonal increases in immunoglobulin, this is closely correlated with age. In studies quoted by

Waldenström[87], a monoclonal immunoglobulin is detectable in 3 per cent of individuals over seventy and 19 per cent in the ninety to ninety-nine decade. Frank multiple myelomatosis is also a disease that increases steadily in incidence with age. A second point of interest is that, of those myeloma proteins that have been identifiable as antibodies, the corresponding antigens have commonly been some body component, often immunoglobulin. Others react with artificial haptens, e.g. dinitrophenyl, which might well be sterically equivalent to certain antigenic determinants on nucleic acids or proteins. Finally, it has already been established that autoantibodies increase in frequency with age, as does the level of total immunoglobulins, and it is well known that most autoimmune diseases are associated with some degree of hypergammaglobulinaemia.

A possible deduction from this set of facts and correlations is that, as the individual ages, somatic mutations, leading eventually to an autoimmune forbidden clone, become more frequent, but the number of cells in which this can occur is probably diminishing rapidly from the exhaustion of stem cells. The combined circumstances would make it more likely that when an autoimmune clone arises it will have the oportunity to develop in monoclonal fashion under stimulation by a more or less ubiquitous body antigen. It must be remembered, too, that a proportion of myelomatoses may be true neoplastic conditions not requiring any antigenic stimulus for their proliferation.

One might conclude that most of the age-association of amyloid disease can be accounted for by a combination of factors: the presence of monoclonal immunoglobulins or fragments thereof in circulation, many with autoimmune implications, plus local accumulations of immunocytes B or T, lethally damaged by a high concentration of antigen or autoantigen whose action is autocatalytically intensified by lymphokines or other products of cell damage. Lest it should be thought that this point of view is more original than it is, it is worth noting that Teilum[88], Briggs[89], Mackay and Burnet[90], and Walford[47] have all previously agreed, in Walford's words, that in amyloidosis 'disturbances in tolerance/homoeostasis/recognition factors, suggestive of autoimmune-like phenomena, are at work'.

CHAPTER 10

ATHEROSCLEROSIS

The most important cause of death in males of the advanced countries of the world is coronary heart disease, with its various synonyms of angina pectoris, heart attack, ischaemic heart disease, or coronary occlusion. This and a substantial proportion of cerebral vascular catastrophes (strokes) result from an arterial disease now usually called atherosclerosis. There is an immense concentration of research on atherosclerosis, and 1969 there was a comprehensive international conference on the topic in Chicago. It has been convenient for me to draw almost everything I am using about atherosclerosis from the reviews and papers in the Conference volume[91], but I am using them for a purpose which is nowhere even suggested in any of the 1969 papers. One would gather that the etiological factors for atherosclerosis were obesity (i.e. over-eating), cigarette smoking, high blood cholesterol, high blood pressure, and emotional tension. No contributor was interested in the genetic side, although it is well known that there is evidence of inheritance of susceptibility to the disease.

A special chapter on atherosclerosis in this book is called for, for three reasons. It is an age-associated disease, as has been already emphasized in the discussion of Burch's theories of autoimmune disease; its lesions are multiple and focal and in the early stages appear to involve cells with a relatively rapid turnover; there is recent work which shows that the initial proliferative lesions in the innermost lining of the large arteries (the intima) have a monoclonal character (see Chapter 4). Perhaps most important of all is the fact that patients with the congenital condition, progeria, who show many signs of premature ageing, usually die of ischaemic heart disease and post mortem show gross atherosclerosis.

Post mortem, early atherosclerosis is seen as discrete foci in the form of raised yellowish areas projecting into the lumen of the aorta and other large arteries. Their number and size increases with advancing age, and in the older lesions there is accumulation of degenerate fatty materials, including cholesterol crystals and phospholipids. More or less impressive imitations of atherosclerosis can be produced by injuring the lining of arteries in rabbits, but the only mammal to develop natural atherosclerotic lesions is the pig. The plaques show a general resemblance to the human lesions and, like them, tend to develop at points of potential turbulence of the blood flow. If the swine are fed a diet high in lipids and have a high blood cholesterol, the atheromatous lesions develop at the preferred sites in a few weeks.

The sites of election in the pig include the trifurcation of the aorta into the two iliac and the caudal arteries. Here in the young animal without lesions there are considerable numbers of separate smooth muscle cells (SMC) in the slightly thickened intima. Appropriate tests with tritiated thymidine show that a fairly rapid cell turnover is taking place. In the developing lesion this appearance is accentuated with the dominant cells SMC, some of which appeared to have de-differentiated towards a fibroblastic appearance and many contain droplets of lipid.

The early human lesions can only be examined post mortem, but in general resemble those of swine with proliferating SMC and usually a continuous one-cell layer of endothelium. Ross *et al.*[(92)] suggest that the SMCs are derived from the endothelium, but this is far from being established. The cells are proliferating and are larger than the few SMCs in unaffected parts of the intima. They are characteristically separated from each other by intercellular matrix of collagen and glycoproteins. Elastin is reduced in amount, or absent. As the lesions become older, they enlarge and may fuse; beneath the superficial fibrous layer the characteristic lipid deposit, including cholesterol crystals and fragments of necrotic cells, develops. Most of the interest of clinicians and biochemists is on the relationship of these deposits to the lipid metabolism of the body, and particularly to blood chloresterol levels. In the light of studies by Benditt and Benditt[(31)], however, the nature of the early proliferative phase overshadows the processes of lipid accumulation and degeneration.

As already mentioned in Chapter 5, these authors have shown that these local proliferations of cells are monoclonal in character.

The material studied came from autopsies of American negro women who were heterozygous A/B for glucose-6-phosphate dehydrogenase (G6PD) and precisely similar technique was used, as in the study of uterine myomas. Electrophoretic detection of A, B or A and B isozymes was possible with extracts from pieces of 1 mm^3 or less. The results were highly significant and, allowing from a small amount of 'noise' from contaminating leucocytes etc., indicated that the cells in each plaque were monoclonal, while in even the smallest fragment possible to test pieces of normal intima showed both A and B. An abbreviated table is shown for the combined results from four individuals.

Table 3 Evidence for the monoclonal character of early atheromatous lesions

Normal intima			*Atherosclerotic plaques*		
AB	A		AB	A	B
57	0	2	6	8	16

The number of small (1 mm^3) pieces of tissue which contained both AB or only a single (A or B) form of the enzyme G6PD are shown. (Data from Benditt and Benditt[31], by courtesy of *Proc. nat. Acad. Sci. U.S.A.*)

Taken at face value, these results can only indicate that each plaque arises as a result of somatic mutation in a single cell with subsequent proliferation of a descendant clone. The Benditts compare the situation to that seen in a myomatous uterus, but it might be a better analogy to compare the early plaque to a freckle or a mole.

There has never been a fully satisfactory interpretation of the initiation of the atheromatous plaque. At the 1969 conference the general opinion seemed to be that some rather subtle form of local damage, probably of hydrodynamic origin, provoked a reparative response. This in turn provides a site where plasma containing lipoproteins etc. could pass into the intima and initiate the lipid infiltration. With the recognition of the monoclonal nature of the initial proliferation, the problem becomes to identify the cell which by mutation found it capable to proliferate in the intimal environment. In view of the capacity of the intima to regenerate very rapidly after injury and the active turnover of endothelial cells, these seem to be likely candidates.

In considering the cause of the mutations the Benditts make the conventional suggestions of an extrinsic agent, either a chemical mutagen or a virus. Both seem extremely unlikely, and if the concept of intrinsic mutagenesis has any validity, here is a situation where it can provide a more satisfying interpretation. In order to offer a specific picture of the situation we can provisionally accept the SMC of the plaque as a mutant form of the endothelial cell which is known to have a rapid turnover, particularly at those sites under hydrodynamic stress where atheroma is most prone to develop. If the SMCs of the intima have some other source than endothelial cells, no serious change is called for.

Any somatic mutation will be most frequent where the number of cell generations is highest. The mutant finds an opportunity to proliferate in the almost acellular substance of the intima, much in the way that mutant melanocytes proliferate to produce a freckle in a red-haired nordic child or a pigment spot on the back of a melanesian albino. The area of local proliferation will be subject to almost the same structural and physiological changes as a minor trauma would produce, and any current interpretation of the processes by which lipid infiltration and various degenerative changes lead to the later 'complicated' stages of atherosclerotic lesions would be equally applicable.

There are several reasons for giving a positive preference to intrinsic mutagenesis as the origin of the multiple somatic mutations to which atherosclerosis is ascribed. In the first place the intima of the aorta is probably the area of the body most completely shielded from any environmental impact and an unprecedented area for virus infection. The multiplicity of foci points necessarily to *somatic* mutation, yet it is strongly suspected that there is an inheritable predisposition to early death from coronary disease. This cannot yet be regarded as definitely established. There is undoubtedly a modest degree of familial association of such deaths, but so many environmental factors are known to play a part that this may be an effect of the family environment (including behavioural aspects) rather than due to genetic causes. Twin studies have in two instances shown a three to five times better concordance of homozygotic as against dizygotic twins, but a third (Danish) study showed no significant difference in this respect. It would be quite unusual if there were no genetic element, but with current techniques it is probably impossible to distinguish the genetic background from the environmental effects.

Even if a clear demonstration of the significance of genetic factors in ischaemic heart disease is achieved, it will still be necessary to allow for the influence of cholesterol blood levels and blood pressure, both of which have genetic components, before claiming a genetic element in the primary atheromatous changes. Any critical experimental study of the latter possibility may well be impossible. It is unlikely that anyone will devise a method of visual examination of the aortic intima in adolescents to determine the number and size of primary atheromatous lesions. However, some less direct method of establishing any genetic significance of the Benditts' discovery may conceivably emerge.

Until the timing and intensity of primary intimal lesions can be shown to be wholly or partly determined genetically, any incrimination of intrinsic mutagenesis in the process must be highly speculative. The age-specific incidence of death from coronary disease has already been mentioned as having a steep straight line curve indicating a cumulative random process strictly related to age. The random episodes involved, however, may involve cells and functions quite unrelated to the postulated initiating lesions. Perhaps the most important evidence of the genetic basis and pathological significance of the primary lesions is the characteristic early death from coronary disease of individuals with progeria.

The origin of the primary atheromatous lesion by intrinsic somatic mutation does not in any way provide a complete etiology for the lethal effects of atherosclerosis. All that could be claimed is that the primary mutational phase is a necessary but not sufficient part of the etiology of what is obviously a highly complex condition. Further study will be needed to establish whether or not lipid concentration in the blood and other adjuvant factors are themselves independently age-associated.

CHAPTER 11

HYPOTHESIS OF THE GENETIC CONTROL OF LIFESPAN

I suspect that for at least thirty years my own philosophy of biology has been essentially that promulgated by Jacques Monod in *Chance and Necessity*[21], but it was never quite at the fully conscious level until I had read his book. Monod's exposition of the nature of life is masterly and irrefutable. Perhaps the essence of his approach is best appreciated in his treatment of the nature of proteins. Each protein, each enzyme, is a polypeptide chain, a sequence made up from twenty different sorts of amino acid. That amino-acid sequence determines everything about the protein, how the polypeptide chain coils and twists to make a three-dimensional molecule, and how, if it is an enzyme, it can recognize and act on its specific substrate. Yet so far there are no rules about sequence. As Monod says, '... even knowing the exact order of 199 residues in a protein containing 200, it would be impossible to formulate any rule, theoretical or empirical, enabling us to predict the nature of the one residue not yet identified by analysis'. In this sense the sequence is a *random* one, and yet it 'is in fact reproduced thousands and thousands of times... by a highly accurate mechanism which guarantees the invariance of the structure'.

Monod is uncompromising in regarding the total organism, even man, as the ultimate expression of the genetic message in the DNA of the zygote and, in one very important sense, nothing else. Change in DNA results only by accident, and, once change has occurred, it is transmitted with the same accuracy as the rest. Acceptance of any such change is by selection for survival. At the level of the whole sexually reproducing organism, the process by which a chance DNA change, initially expressed in one individual, is accepted or not into the whole or a significant portion of the population that makes up a species is too complex for discussion here. Selection for survival is, however, a much simpler process when we are concerned with body cells modified by somatic mutation in which only dominant or co-dominant changes can be expressed.

Monod has virtually nothing to say in *Chance and Necessity* about the ecology and evolution of somatic cells within the body, but his basic principles obviously apply. If there is, to use Monod's phrase, a teleonomic necessity for some structural or functional adaptation to new requirements, it can be reached only by a random process, which is then tested for survival by selection at some appropriate level. The nature of antibody production is a particularly good example at the somatic cell level.

Here the basic requirement was that the body should have available cells which could react specifically with foreign material of unknown and unknowable chemical structure entering the body usually as a result of microorganismal infection. To oversimplify but still present the essence of the problem we can say that the cells secrete a protein (antibody) which attaches specifically to the microorganism and facilitates its destruction by phagocytosis. It is equally important that the body should preserve a *memory* of how the infection was overcome and retain representatives of the cell clones that were involved. For the persistence of memory in those cells the only possible repository of the information is DNA. If antibodies with this character of memory are to be available, the only possible way of producing them is to allow accelerated random processes to occur in an appropriate gene or group of genes which will ensure that a wide enough range of antibody patterns is produced to cover perhaps 90 per cent, perhaps 99 per cent, of the infections or other emergencies which may call for an immune response. As Jerne(93) has pointed out, on simple stochastic principles random processes can never provide 100 per cent effectiveness in any function. The number of potential antibody patterns that *could* be produced by the species is bound to be many times larger than the actual number produced by any individual. It is equally axiomatic that no two individuals will develop the same detailed pattern of immune response.

Details of how these 'repertoires' of immune pattern are generated are still basically unknown. A few workers believe that all the alternatives are individually controlled by germ-line genes that have been accumulated over the whole period of mammalian evolution. This is hardly compatible with the wide range of distinguishable antibodies observed when the individual responses of a group of pure-line mice immunized with the same antigen are compared. A majority of immunologists assume that a limited range of patterns is transmitted in the germ line and that randomizing processes take place in embryonic stem cells, so that by the time of birth a significant fraction of the possible repertoire is available. There are at least two quite distinct ways in which one can picture how such randomization can happen.

The process of phenotypic restriction by which only one type of antibody pattern is expressed in cells of any one clone has a number of analogies in other forms of cellular differentiation but is still to be adequately explained at the molecular level. Despite all the controversy, however, there is no significant support anywhere for the old instructive theories by which antigen stamped a complementary pattern on the newly synthesized immunoglobulin. Such a view is now unthinkable; it conflicts flatly with the two dogmas of molecular biology which are basic to all thought about living process. The first is that information moves from DNA to protein and never in the opposite direction, and the second, that the amino-acid sequence of a polypeptide chain uniquely determines the three-dimensional configuration that it will adopt.

The significance of somatic mutation

The possibility that much the same principles that underlie the theory of clonal selection in immunity could be applied to the problems of malignant disease and ageing has been germinating in my mind since at least 1957. In a sense, the somatic mutation theory of cancer, which in various guises has been current for many years, was an adequate model. Unfortunately it had no bearing on the obvious relationship in all mammalian species between the time of ageing and the accompanying upsurge of cancer incidence. What was needed was some hypothesis which would allow the genome to control the average lifespan so as to ensure that ageing takes place at a time appropriate to the life style of the species and at the same time offer a reason for the strictly age-associated incidence of nearly all cancers. More recently I have become increasingly aware of the equally important need to understand the age-associated focal and general degenerative diseases of the central nervous system.

In this chapter I attempt to describe in more detail the hypothesis foreshadowed in the introduction and forming a central theme in the book, that the genetic control of ageing, more specifically the length of the average lifespan, is based on the 'goodness of fit' of enzymes concerned with the primary functions of the genetic mechanism.

Investigation of the structure of the RNA of a small RNA bacteriophage—the simplest genome yet available—reveals that there are sequences of nucleotides beyond those coding for all the functional proteins. In bacteria and in higher organisms it is necessary to postulate functions mediated by nucleotide segments or genes other than the structural genes directly concerned with protein synthesis. Their functions are largely unknown, but presumably they are concerned wholly with activities within the genome itself. It is possible that opinions may change, but at the present time I know of no suggestion that the genome has any influence on the somatic structure of the body that is not mediated through the linear specification of the primary protein chains. The dogma that the tertiary structure of a protein is implicit in the linear arrangement of the component amino-acid residues is now well established. Most of the proteins specified by any genome are enzymes, and by hypothesis all the functions of each enzyme molecule are specified by its linear sequence of amino-acid residues and by that alone. This carries the fantastic implication that the simple linear configuration of an enzyme molecule carries the information needed to ensure that in the intracellular environment it takes on its appropriate three-dimensional form, finds its functionally appropriate position in some cellular organelle, and also provides specific patterns that allow other relevant macromolecules to coordinate their activities with its own. It is often the case that an enzyme, particularly one concerned with the first stage of metabolic sequence, is specifically reactive with another molecule than its substrate. This is usually the end product of the sequence, and as a result of union the configuration of the enzyme-binding site is distorted and its activity turned off. This is the 'allosteric inhibition' of Monod and Jacob; it represents just one more aspect of the specific 'information' built into the enzyme by the sequence of its amino-acid residues.

One can never wholly exclude the possibility that there is some additional mode by which the genome controls cellular function other than through the qualities endowed on proteins by their amino-acid sequences. Hahn[94] has raised the possibility that ageing is associated with functional impairment of intranuclear regulatory processes, perhaps located in the association of histone with nucleic acid. Even in such a case, however, the quality of the histone is in the last analysis under DNA control. I can see no alternative to the conclusion that the nexus between an information-bearing sequence of nucleotides in DNA and length of lifespan must be sought in the properties of one or more proteins.

The seminal idea in this field seems to be Orgel's error catastrophe hypothesis[45] which has been mentioned earlier (see page 60). This assumes that error (mutation) in key enzymes, such as those concerned in any of the essential steps of transcription or translation by which nuclear information is expressed in the pattern of proteins will necessarily lead eventually to a catastrophic pile-up of errors, involving many different enzymes. This must hold also, particularly for cell lines subject to continuous clonal proliferation, if structural anomalies appear in the enzymes which play a part in the accurate replication of DNA. From our point of view the role of DNA polymerase is the crucial one.

The evidence from bacterial genetics referred to earlier has indicated the necessity for a high degree of fidelity in the duplication of DNA and in its repair after damage. Any accumulation of errors beyond a certain level will render a potential clone non-viable, but equally, unless an occasional error is possible, evolutionary change stops completely. Every enzyme has evolved to coordinate sterically with its substrate molecule and any other associated enzymes or smaller molecules that are relevant to its catalytic function. Complex steric interactions of this sort will demand an optimal and constant structure of the enzyme molecule. Any replacement of one amino-acid residue by another will by hypothesis diminish the effectiveness of enzymic action. In principle, an infinite range of modification of 'goodness of fit' could be introduced by mutational changes in the sequence. To give an indication of the influence of mutation on enzyme function a specific example may be examined.

In discussing the results of somatic proliferation and its bearing on the monoclonal origin of some disease conditions, I had occasion to mention the enzyme commonly known as G6PD (glucose-6-phosphate dehydrogenase) as an index of monoclonality. This enzyme[95] has probably been more widely studied in regard to its range of genetic variability than any other and therefore offers a particularly suitable example of how an enzyme can be modified by mutation. G6PD in its normal form is concerned at a vital point in the chain of reactions that oxidize glucose to lactic acid in the body. Its clinical importance is that if it is not functioning adequately in the red cell, the cell membrane becomes unstable, allowing loss of haemoglobin and, depending on circumstances, either an acute or a chronic haemolytic anaemia.

The existence of abnormal forms of G6PD was first recognized by the occurrence of severe haemolytic anaemia in negro servicemen in the United States army who were being given anti-malarial drugs. It soon became evident that only a proportion of male negroes were susceptible to this drug-induced haemolytic anaemia and that the susceptibility was a genetic trait. The structural gene responsible is carried on the X chromosome and research to date has uncovered eighty different variants of the enzyme corresponding to eighty different allelic forms of the gene. In all probability, most of the variants represent changes in a single amino-acid residue, although this has so far been experimentally established for only three of them.

The variants are distinguished by the kinetics of their catalytic action, by their electrophoretic behaviour, and by their range of substrates. Clinically, the eighty alleles can be divided into three groups:

1. About forty, including the two common, normal forms (A^+, mainly in negroes, and B^+), have normal, or only slightly diminished, activity and cause no symptoms.
2. There are some twenty alleles (including the classic A^-, responsible for most of the haemolytic anaemias in negroes given anti-malarial drugs) in which some triggering agent—drug, an acute infection, or certain foods, notably broad beans (favism)—is needed to provoke haemolysis.
3. In a final group, again of about twenty alelles, a chronic haemolytic anaemia is produced without the necessity for any exogenous agent.

There are many interesting details of these eighty forms of a single enzyme, but they are quite irrelevant in the present context. What is important is that we have here a well studied example of the degree to which genetic modification of an enzyme can cocur and still allow the organism to function. There may well be a much greater number of possible mutations which are never recognized because they prevent any functioning of the enzyme and are therefore lethal to the embryo. One can reasonably assume that most or all other enzymes in the body are similarly subject to mutational changes. There are ninety-one clinical disorders that are recognized as due to a genetically deficient enzyme, and it seems to be invariable that when any such deficiency disease is common enough to allow comprehensive study, several varieties of deficient enzyme are found.

If we accept the dogma that *all* verifiably genetic diseases are due directly or indirectly to abnormal structure in one or more enzymes, there must be enormously greater number of pathogenically active enzyme variants. In a 1971 compilation[96] there are said to be 415 accepted types of autosomal dominant abnormality plus another 528 possibles that are so far inadequately studied. For autosomal recessives the count is 365 established and 418 possibles, and for X-linked conditions 86, plus 64 still in question.

The whole function of this interlude is to establish the legitimacy of hypotheses ascribing biological phenomena to mutations—either germ-line or somatic—resulting in structural change and functional deficiency in an enzyme. Clearly it is within the potentialities of the genome to produce a range of molecular variants of any enzyme which can cover the whole range of accuracy of fit or effectiveness of function. Error in a proportion of end products of some complex and coordinated process, whether molecules, cells, or industrial products, is always tolerable, but error in the 'design stages' can be fatal since it is reflected in *all* the products. Orgel pictured the result of a mutation which significantly reduced the effectiveness of any enzyme that had a share in responsibility for the accuracy of the processes of transcription and translation needed to ensure the correct transfer of information from DNA to protein. Even more important for continuously proliferating cells would be any failure to produce accurate replicas of the DNA itself, which would introduce secondary errors into the structure of proteins controlled by the DNA segments in which error had occurred. Any enzyme in the body or in a cell clone, depending on whether the initial mutation was in the germ-line or somatic, could become subject to error and dysfunction. In principle all enzymes could be regarded as being equally likely to suffer such mutational distortion, including the enzymes concerned with the accuracy of DNA-, RNA- and protein-synthesis. Whenever one of these is involved, the situation is automatically worsened. Eventually a cascading situation would develop, with a runaway build-up of non-functioning or malfunctioning enzymes throughout the cell—an error catastrophe. If no other factors intervened, such a process would eventually involve all the cells of the clone concerned, the time or the number of cell generations required being a function of the degree of error-proneness of the initial replicating enzyme system.

In principle, evolution could adjust the specification, say, of a DNA-polymerase characteristic of the immunicyte, at any level needed to produce a desirable level of somatic mutability, and in this way to determine the time after development had begun when a cell line would be most likely to break down in an error catastrophe. Basically similar principles could apply to the non-multiplying post-mitotic cells of the central nervous system or to any other cell system of the body. Average lifespan is determined by the rate at which inefficiency of function and vulnerability to disease develops, something which can be looked at as an integration of the various patterns of error catastrophe and cell death throughout the body.

In all this we are primarily concerned with the processes which determine the average lifespan in essentially normal individuals. It must, however, be equally evident that on occasion mutation involving the same group of genes may induce a pathological level of error-proneness in a key enzyme. In such individuals one could expect to find genetic anomalies associated either with general acceleration of ageing or focal degenerative changes. Discussion of this aspect will be deferred to Chapters 16 and 17; here we are dealing only with the normal process of ageing.

If the Hayflick limit is a result of an accumulation of somatic mutations whose frequency is governed by the structure of a DNA polymerase (or some other enzyme necessary for the accurate replication of DNA pattern), and if the Hayflick limit in its turn is largely responsible for the timing of the process of senescene, we have at least a possible path from DNA structure to the characteristic lifespan of each species. It remains to look for evidence that can be used to support or to oppose an hypothesis of this general character.

The Hayflick limit

In Hayflick's original work with human fibroblast cell cultures he suggested that the fall-off in cell numbers had the quality of a multi-hit curve and could represent the effect of numerous somatic mutations. A direct approach, involving a search for abnormal enzymes in fibroblast cultures approaching their limit of growth, has been made successfully by Holliday and Tarrant(97) and by Lewis and Tarrant(98). They studied three enzymes (glucose-6-phosphate dehydrogenase, 6-phosphogluconate dehydrogenase, and lactose dehydrogenase) and examined changes in the heat stability of the enzyme or the changing ratio between the concentration of enzyme assessed immunologically and functionally. Immunological identification of an enzyme will not usually differentiate between the normal functional enzyme and defective mutants. Fully active enzyme will give a certain standard ratio between the two measurements, but any significant deficiency in enzymatic function will change the ratio. A progressive fall in the ratio of functional activity to the amount of enzyme assayed immunologically indicates the accumulation of mutant enzyme protein. By both methods there was a sharp increase in altered enzyme in the last ten generations of cell growth as fibroblasts approached the Hayflick limit.

Similar changes have been found by the use of 5-fluor-deoxyuridine to produce premature senescence of the cultures. In earlier work by Holliday[(99)], amino-acid analogues, which would also result in the appearance of altered enzymes, produced premature ageing in fungal cultures. Various authors have observed losses of enzymic activity in ageing cell cultures. Goldstein and Singal[(100)] found that in some, but not all, human fibroblast clones approaching the Hayflick limit the HL-A histocompatibility antigens were lost.

All this work is consistent with an Orgel-type explanation but is hardly sufficient to establish it. However, in the absence of any alternative explanation and its general 'biological reasonableness' I shall provisionally adopt it.

The next step in this more technical examination of the basic hypothesis has to do with the relevance of the Hayflick limit to situations in the body. A cell in culture is a very incomplete entity, biologically speaking, compared to a functioning cell in the living organism. Even if the principles of a limit hold in the body, its manifestations may be much more difficult to demonstrate. There are, for instance, very long-lived lymphocytes in circulation which may persist without multiplication for several years, and any sample of fibroblasts is certain to be polyclonal and to contain cells with widely differing distances from the zygote in terms of all generations. One could not, therefore, expect to find that the Hayflick limit of fibroblasts from, say, human tissues of individuals from infancy to old age should show an accurately proportional fall in the number of available cell generations with age. Martin *et al.*[(49)], however, showed a fairly regular negative regression on the age of the donor for the Hayflick limit, from forty-five cell generations for foetal tissue to twenty-six for donors from eight to eighty-five. It may be significant that the lowest number for the eighty to eighty-five was eight cell generations for bone marrow cells. There are a number of syndromes, presumably genetic in origin, which are associated with premature ageing. One of these is Werner's syndrome[(101)] in which the mean age of death is forty-seven and more than 10 per cent of patients die of malignant disease. Fibroblasts from such a patient survived only five to six cell generations in culture.

Of even more interest are the findings recently reported for progeria[(102)].

This is a congenital condition in which the child develops many of the standards signs of old age and at seven or nine years looks like 'a frail, little old man'. The average age at death is about fourteen years and the longest survival on record twenty-seven years.

Fibroblasts from skin of such patients are difficult to initiate in cell culture and, once established, last for a greatly restricted number of generations, about eleven. The most important anomaly of these cells is, however, their inability to repair DNA broken by heavy X-irradiation. This was measured by an *in vitro* method in which normal human fibroblasts repaired broken DNA completely in thirty minutes, while under the same conditions progeroid cells showed only a trace of repair after 270 minutes.

In an earlier chapter I have given a simplified version of Williamson and Askonas's[44] demonstration of the limited number of cell generations that are available to an established clone of antibody-producing cells. This was no surprise to immunologists as there had been much earlier work using radioisotope labelling which indicated that an active plasma cell line persisted for only eight to ten generations after its first appearance in plasma cell form.

Complexities of the situation

The doubts that have been expresed by Franks, Walford and others about the general applicability of the Hayflick limit have been referred to on several occasions already. Their attitude is broadly that, until the Hayflick phenomenon in human cell cultures is more adequately shown to result from error catastrophe of mutational origin and not from some inadequacy of the technique, it is dangerous to use it for so crucial a point in a theory of ageing. The main reason for so using it has of course been the promise it gave of connecting the run-down of thymic function with a genetically determined level of somatic mutation. The joint concept of error catastrophe and Hayflick limit is the most readily visible way by which a genetically defined capacity for error can be expressed to provide an intermediary step toward the achievement of an appropriate lifespan. Everything seems to fit neatly together, but one's general experience of biology says insistently that reality must be much more complex than this.

In my proper discipline of immunology, analysis of a complex functional system has probably gone as deep as anywhere in biology. What has emerged from two decades of intensive research is not a clear picture.

Influenced by some of Jerne's recent writings, I have expressed the present day situation of immunological research as trying to make sense of two-dimensional sections of a multi-dimensional probabilistic network. The relevant parameters become more and more numerous each year; more interactions between cell types or between cells and soluble substances are observed and investigated and most quantitative experiments give a soft-edged result. In a field of my own special interest —tolerance and immunosuppression, including the anomalies that present as autoimmune disease—the complexities seem to have become endless. I find myself speaking of fail-safe systems and look forward without enthusiasm to a system that is not only a complexly interacting network, but has also some aspects of the cascade structure of the blood-clotting mechanism and almost certainly a similar collection of inhibitors and feedback controls.

Immunology deals with one aspect of differentiation, which for technical and historical reasons has proved to be more amenable to scientific study than any other aspect of mammalian function. It is axiomatic, for me at least, that every other aspect of mammalian differentiation will have its own multi-dimensional network of interactions as complex as anything we have found in the immune system. No one has even suggested how, if ever, the whole process of differentiation from the zygote to the adult mammal will become expressible in molecular terms. To attempt to understand the breakdown of differentiation —which is ageing—can be only marginally simpler. Obviously the minimal requirement is an understanding of the functional and structural homoeostasis of the mature animal, including the processes of repair of non-lethal damage of various sorts. However, the possibility of obtaining useful general ideas by studying the behaviour of a biological system which has been 'damaged' in various definable ways, genetically, pharmacologically or surgically, has been exemplified in many areas of medical research. In a number of instances a genetic lesion has been most illuminating for normal physiology, e.g. agammaglobulinaemia, colour blindness, haemophilia, and alkaptonuria.

If the present approach to ageing is to be criticized, the most obvious (and irrefutable) objection will be that the process of senescene is a highly complex one and that any attempt to concentrate attention on the genetically controlled rate of somatic mutation is bound to be inadequate. At least a partial answer is to claim that observed complexity of effect does not exclude the whole result being primarily dependent on a simple primary situation. If there is a basic function which determines lifespan it is necessarily exerted with a highly complex interrelated system and will inevitably produce a diversity of secondary effects. What seems to be inescapable is that cell lines accumulate mutations as indicated by enzyme inadequacies, loss of histocompatibility antigens etc. If, as everything suggests, the process is a random one informationally, a very wide range of changes will soon be found in any clonally proliferating population. The demonstrable effect, whether in the form of a Hayflick limit or enzyme ineffeciency in the laboratory, or as a tissue atrophy or abnormal proliferation *in vivo*, will depend greatly on the cell line and the circumstances.

In discussing the part played by immunocyte lines, insufficient emphasis may have been laid on the greater scope for mutation to produce changed reactivity in these cells than in any other somatic cells. In particular, one must postulate great potentiality for change in the type and degree of response of a cell to contact with antigenic determinants capable of significant interaction with the specific receptors of the immunocyte. Under normal conditions a considerable range of responses, proliferative, inhibitory, or productive of lymphokines, can take place. Somatic mutation could, in principle, allow changed reactivities of various degrees which could be expressed either in minor immunological anomalies or more grossly pathological conditions, from frank lymphosarcoma to leukaemia, myelomatosis, and autoimmune disease. Accelerated destruction of immunocytes reacting with antigen is the most likely interpretation of amyloid deposition. Any of these might occur in addition to the error catastrophe postulated from analogy with fibroblast cultures.

In other proliferating cell lines the effect of error accumulation will depend on circumstances. On the whole, Krohn's serial transplantation experiments[(103)] point to a slow ageing of the skin although it survives two to three times the maximum lifespan of the animal. It seems by no means necessary nor likely that the available cell generations should be exhausted at approximately the same time in each tissue. It is clear enough from human experience that death is in the great majority a random episode, often a vascular mishap in an organism that has become vulnerable but for the most part is still functionally effective. Death that can be ascribed to simple senility is exceedingly rare.

Ascription of thymic atrophy to exhaustion of cell generations may be correct, but most pathologists would feel that this may be much more a matter of programmed development than of atrophy from a variable and essentially random using up of a quota of cells. In view of the intense susceptibility of the bursa of Fabricius to inhibition by testosterone and related steroids and its disappearance at sexual maturity, a substantial part of the initial diminution in thymus weight at puberty must be assigned to hormonal effects and be regarded as part of a genetic programme. Once the adolescent phase is over, however, further atrophy has most of the attributes of a random fade-out. In other tissues, too, programmed responses to hormonal and other stimuli will continue until the changes resulting from any type of sequential error make them impossible. Only the cells of an exceptionally malignant tumour have lost all responsiveness to the controls responsible for internal homoeostasis.

Age changes in non-proliferating cells

In view of the important part in human ageing of cerebral and mental deterioration, in a tissue whose cells are all post-mitotics incapable of replication, concentration wholly on clonally proliferating cells must be quite inadequate. Curtis's work on the liver also suggests that age-related changes in cells can develop in the virtual absence of proliferation. At the present time there is great interest in but no clear explanation of the existence in vertebrate cells of multiple copies of certain DNA segments. Pelc[(104)] regarded this as possibly related to the small uptake of thymidine by the nuclei of post-mitotic cells in the brain or elsewhere. On this view, 'working' DNA is in the form of copies of a master gene and its metabolic activity represents either repair of damage arising in the course of transcription to m RNA or replacement by replication. Irrespective of whether 'master' or 'slave' DNA units were involved, the accumulating errors would concern especially those enzymes and other proteins that need constant renewal in the cell. This would not lead to error catastrophe but could slowly diminish functional activity and perhaps be responsible for the alleged progresisve disappearance of single neurones in the brain over most of life. Clearly the enzymes concerned in these cells must be repair DNA polymerases rather than replicases, that is if the two functions can be effectively separated.

A point raised by Curtis[(48)] may be mentioned here. He was impressed that treatment of mice with up to LD50 doses of nitrogen-mustard allowed the appearance of a variety of chromosomal damage in circulating lymphocytes, but the survivors showed no significant shortening of lifespan. In his view, damage to actively proliferating cells can be rapidly nullified by elimination of the damaged cells and their replacement by new ones. This point may be legitimately applied to cells with multiple damage by nitrogen-mustard and similar agents, but is not necessarily relevant to mutations initiated by intrinsic processes. With cells of the immunocyte series, mutational changes are as likely to remove susceptibility to controls inhibiting or disintegrating the cells as to render the cells incapable of normal proliferation. The increasing frequency of autoantibodies with age is the prototype of this.

Programmed deterioration as alternative

It is accepted in every discussion of ageing that the average lifespan of every mammalian group is genetically programmed. In principle there are only two mechanisms by which the programme could be implemented; they may be briefly identified as error accumulation and programmed deterioration.

The first is what the present hypothesis has been concerned with. By programmed deterioration one imagines a development analogous, say, to puberty, by which at some key signal, a change in the balance of circulating pituitary and other hormones perhaps, a large range of cells swing into a 'suicidal' phase. Medvedev spoke of the possibility of their being programmed to respond to such a stimulus by bringing nonsense genes into action. A more acceptable possibility would be to suggest that at this hypothetical trigger phase of ageing a new set of DNA polymerases with genetically inbuilt capacity for a high level of mutagenesis was swung into action to replace the accurate enzymes of youth and maturity. The analogy here might be with the switch from foetal to standard haemoglobin around the time of birth.

There is nothing biologically impossible in the concept that at some appropriate stage a maximally efficient DNA repair enzyme should be replaced by one with a built-in capacity to generate errors. Intuitively this interpretation seems both unattractive and unlikely. In the first place its implementation would require a complex chain of events, including a timing mechanism about which we have not even a suggestion as to its site or quality. A more significant objection is the difficulty of stating the time at which ageing begins. In all probability it is a progressively accelerating process which may start at conception and in man is certainly detectable from the age of twenty onward. Apart from the female menopause, there is no evident break in the progress of normal ageing that could coincide with the switching-on of an alternative set of error-prone enzymes. An accumulation of errors over the whole lifespan makes much better sense, provided one remembers that any attempt to pinpoint one dominant factor for some general biological function, such as growth, repair, malignant disease, or ageing, will always require that the factor be integrated with and modify or be modified by any or all of the other aspects of the living organism and the evolving species concerned.

Our central thesis can only be understood if it is clearly recognized that if the hypothesis of cumulative error in the action of key enzymes is even partly correct there must be adjustments at two levels. Any significant shortening or lengthening of the lifespan of a *species* called for by some ecological change must necessarily be associated with an appropriate restructuring of the consecutive compartments of mammalian life, gestation, immaturity, reproductive maturity, senescence and death. How this is achieved lies outside our field, but we know, for example by comparing different domestic breeds of dogs, that it is within the capacity of selective breeding or natural evolution. In a broadly equivalent fashion any modification of lifespan in an *individual*, whether by genetic or other influences, will have repercussions on the incidence of various age-associated conditions. Some interesting examples were observed in McCay's rats[64] whose lives were prolonged by balanced under-nutrition in the post-weaning period.

Possibly the most important point to be made in this discussion of difficulties is that the postulated source of a slowly mounting accumulation of errors must work within a pattern of normal homoeostasis and that changes resulting from error will set in progress any counteracting processes incorporated in the homoeostatic repertoire of the body. In one way and another, the expression of error will largely be nullified in earlier life and become more and more evident in later life as the homeostatic mechanisms themselves become prone to error.

A new paradigm

Any survey of the current status of research and speculation on the nature of ageing is likely to provoke two main impressions: first, that there must be some fundamental and probably rather simple basis for the evident regularities of the process, and second, the great diversity of the means of age-associated death and the obviously random character of many of the processes at work. It is possible that the simple interpretative summary given by Cutler[105] is as far as it is legitimate to go. He considered that for each species there is a specific genetic programme for the characteristic lifespan. Random errors which progressively damage metabolic processes, but at rates varying with the individual, modify the programme to give the familiar Gompertz-type survival curves.

Something more than this is needed and one senses that most gerontologists feel that the time is, or soon will be, ripe for the introduction of a new type of scientific approach to their field—a new paradigm in terms of T. S. Kuhn's *Structure of Scientific Revolutions*[106]. Kuhn's approach seems to be equally relevant, whether the changes are the great steps of Newton, Planck and Einstein with which Kuhn is mainly concerned or some quite unimportant change of approach to a minor biological field. The essential feature of a scientific revolution is that within the field, large or small, that is involved, a new general approach, a new paradigm is called for which will in due course, if it is useful and successful, change the character of 'normal' experimental science that is appropriate in the field.

There can be no question that the conjoint field of ageing, degenerative disease, and cancer is not at present covered by any paradigm in Kuhn's sense. The nearest approach is the concentration of experimental cancer research into a paradigm analogous to that which has been so successful in elucidating the molecular biology of the interactions of *E. coli* and its bacteriophages, in essence that cancer represents one of the results of the intrusion of viral nucleic acid into a somatic cell genome. At a number of earlier points I have indicated what seem to be major objections to this approach. The most important is the almost complete irrelevance of the experimental work to the problem it is supposed to be concerned with, the common lethal cancers of human beings. This weakness of current 'normal science' as applied to malignant disease is quite evidently a crisis in Kuhn's sense.

The whole of the present discussion can be regarded as part of a process aimed at a new paradigm relevant to the scientific study of senescence and malignant disease. It is something that has been under way for at least twenty years and so far its most effective approach has been by the application of stochastic mathematical methods to the data of the incidence of cancer. Examples that may be mentioned include the work of Armitage and Doll[107], P. R. J. Burch[40], and Knudson and Strong[108]. All of these have been concerned with human material. Research on animal lifespans is not an immediately rewarding occupation. Very large numbers of animals are necessary, meticulous husbandry must be maintained for long periods, and any accidental infection may ruin years of work. It is unlikely that any laboratory will ever produce experimental animal material or spontaneous neoplasia that will be of equivalent magnitude and quality to the best human statistics.

All the statistical work depends on some stochastic interpretation to cover a random process whose biological nature imposes certain rules. In practice the interpretation has always been in terms of a random process or a sequence of such processes with a definable frequency in terms of nucleotide, gene, nucleus, or individual, on the one hand, and time or generation, on the other. In the specific field of cancer initiation the only process available is somatic mutation. We are necessarily concerned with events which are rare, which involve a single cell, and whose effect is evident in all descendants of the initially influenced cell. Those features define somatic mutation.

It follows that eventual acceptance of what might be called the paradigm of somatic mutation in relation to ageing and neoplastic disease will necessarily deflect experimental research or cancer into a new direction—into channels that bear on the nature and stochastic origin of somatic mutation. The whole central thesis of this discussion, that somatic mutation is not due to thermal agitation, background radiation or some other purely physical factor, but to a biologically significant and measurably infidelity of DNA replication, may be completely wrong. Even if there is no biological reason in somatic mutation, the experimental steps to disprove the hypothesis of intrinsic mutagenesis are the same as those needed to establish its implications and limitations if it should be proved to be partly true and experimentally productive. Analysis of the enzymes concerned with replication and repair of DNA in mammalian cells is not in principle different from what has already been done in great detail for *E. coli* and bacteriophage T4. The fact that a gene coding for DNA polymerase can, on mutation, function as a mutator or anti-mutator gene for T4 is the key finding on which the hypothesis is built. It would be wholly in line with the history of biochemistry and genetics that a clue to the nature of ageing and cancer should first be sought in *E. coli* and its viruses. To define the structural differences in T4 DNA polymerases, which determine their error-producing potential, would seem to be the first experimental approach towards defining intrinsic mutagenesis. Until this or some equivalent study at viral or bacterial level is achieved, work with mammalian cells will probably have to be at a fairly superficial level. What has already been established for cells from the genetic diseases, progeria, Werner's syndrome, and xeroderma pigmentosum, however, indicates the potentialities of relatively simple studies. At least there can be no objection to the hypothesis on the ground that it cannot be disproved by experimental methods that are currently practicable.

I believe, too, that the requirement implicit in Monod's philosophy—and mine—that the problem of the nexus between an evolutionary requirement and its achievement must be solved in a random fashion moulded by selection, is more reasonably filled by an hypothesis of this general type than by any alternative yet put forward.

PART 3

Malignant Disease

CHAPTER 12

MALIGNANT DISEASE—1

Cancer is not the most frequent cause of death in old age, but it is the most feared, and more than any other disease of the old it has had a perennial fascination for both pathologist and philosopher as something basically unreasonable and therefore a challenge to understanding. Here I am concerned primarily in seeking a reason for the characteristic association of cancer with ageing in every species for which information is available.

With a few important exceptions, all forms of malignant disease become progressively more frequent with age. If one takes all deaths from cancer and plots them according to age groups in terms of the number of cases per annum per 10 000 people alive in the age group concerned, the line rises steadily with age. If the scales on both coordinates are logarithmic, the graph is extremely close to a straight line. This line suggests that if people escaped all other causes of death indefinitely, they would *all* die of cancer by the time they were 150 years old! More importantly, the regularity of the curve indicates that overall there are some almost universal processes at work in determining the incidence of cancer in relation to age.

At the present time there is probably near unanimity that, provided one accepts any abrupt change in a cell which is indefinitely transmitted to the cells of its descendant clone, as somatic mutation, all malignant tumours result from the occurrence of somatic mutation, and particularly of sequences of mutations which may include germ-line components. Difference of opinion arises when the *cause* of the somatic mutation is considered. As has already emerged at several points, the predominant view is that mutations represent random damage to DNA by chemical agents, radiation, or non-destructive infection by viruses; many would add wholly random changes in DNA, presumably due to thermal molecular agitation. If the hypothesis of intrinsic mutagenesis is to be extended to cover the phenomena of malignancy, the role of these causes of mutation will need to be modified significantly. Like the more direct manifestations of senescence, we shall regard cancer as induced mainly by the accumulation of error in DNA duplication and repair due to infidelity in the functioning of DNA polymerases and the other enzymes concerned. Not every cancer that is induced reaches full clinical expression. There is adequate evidence that cellular changes which would otherwise lead to cancer can be checked (*a*) by maturation of embryonal cell tumours such as neuroblastoma, and (*b*) by immune responses to abnormal antigens carried by the changed cells.

Since 1957 I have consistently supported the view that somatic mutation is responsible for the essential change that bestows on the cancer cell and its descendants the characteristic capacity for inadequately controlled growth[(109)]. Extrinsic cancer-provoking agents, physical, chemical or viral, were regarded essentially as mutagens. In the present attempt to reach a more satisfactory interpretation both the intrinsic and the extrinsic factors will need to be scrutinized.

The environmental causes of cancer are more amenable to study than its 'spontaneous' occurrence and there is an immense literature on the experimental induction of cancer by polycyclic hydrocarbons, from tar in the first instance, and subsequently by a very wide range of organic chemicals. Equally active investigation followed the discovery in the early years of the century that excessive exposure to X-rays or radium could induce cancer, and in recent years the greatest concentration of cancer research has been on the role of viruses as causes of cancer in experimental animals and possibly in man. All three types of agent will need discussion, but it is convenient to reverse the order and begin with the relation of viruses to malignant disease.

'Cancer viruses'

In human experience no forms of malignant disease have been indubitably produced by a virus and there is no fully accepted evidence that there is any possibility of malignant disease being transmissible from one person to another. Many workers, however, would probably claim that, though the evidence is incomplete, the balance of probabilities is that childhood leukaemia will eventually be accepted as a very rare manifestation of some common infection. Infectious mononucleosis (glandular fever) is a possible candidate for the role. Others would go much further and assume that all human cancers are more or less disguised manifestations of non-cytotoxic viral infection, of which the well studied tumours that can be produced by viruses in mice and chickens provide a model. The investigation of human tumours for viruses by classical methods of isolation has been quite unsuccessful except for those exotic tumours, Burkitt's lymphoma and nasopharyngeal carcinoma, which are dealt with in Chapter 15. The modern approach to human cancer virology is more sophisticated and indirect, involving recognition in the cells of cultured tumours, either antigens cross-reacting with viral antigens or DNA that will 'hybridize' with nucleic acid from virus-induced animal tumours. My own minority opinion is that most or all of the results of this work will find other interpretations, of which those suggested by Temin[(110)] (the protovirus hypothesis) or by Dulbecco may be forerunners.

Amongst recent discussion of the field, I find the most balanced and acceptable approach in Dulbecco's 1973 Marjory Stephenson lecture[(110a)]. As I understand it, he believes that the oncogenic activity of polyoma (DNA) viruses is a more or less accidental by-product, with no evolutionary importance, of the process common to all viruses of intrusion of viral genome into that of the host cell. This is 'designed' to allow viral multiplication, death of the cell, and release of the virus to infect another host. Nothing else is significant at the level of evolution of the virus. By simple accident, some cells are not so influenced; intrusion into the host genome of such non-permissive cells results in integration of the whole or portions of the virus genome into that of the host, but the complete take-over is not achieved. Instead, the viral genetic material is passively carried without harm to the cell in the great majority of instances. In a proportion, however, one of the incorporated virus genes induces a change in the cell which with some simplification is shown as 'transformation' in culture and malignancy *in vivo* under the right conditions. In this way, what can be called a transforming gene has been identified in the virus genome but with the necessary reservation that its 'real' evolutionary function is to allow virus proliferation and liberation from a permissive cell.

Dulbecco's analysis of the leukovirus situation is almost completely parallel to my own intuitive reaction, but is based on a much deeper understanding of the technical details. He divides the leukoviruses into two classes. The first contains the sarcoma viruses, characteristically variants which have arisen in the laboratory from less active agents; these transform all the cells they infect and possess a 'transforming gene'. The second group of leukoviruses are very widespread but, except in some genetically unusual hosts, transform only a minute proportion of the cells they infect. They possess no transforming gene, and in Dulbecco's words 'can only transform cells in which the cellular gene balance is altered in a certain way by rare virus-independent events'. I should substitute 'by somatic mutation' for the last phrase. Dulbecco suggests that the sarcoma viruses have arisen in laboratories from defective leukoviruses which have been reconstituted by incorporation of a segment from some other genome, possibly from a DNA virus-like polyoma. A sarcoma virus, in his view, is an 'unnatural virus . . . perpetuated by the experimenter who supplies the selective advantage denied by nature'. Such viruses have no possible relevance to age-associated human cancer and no further attempt will be made to discuss their significance.

The herpesviruses typified by EBV are of much greater interest. They have been extensively investigated and have an established relationship to at least three clinically significant conditions. As there are aspects of this group which are relevant to our specific interest in the age-association of malignant disease, a fairly detailed discussion of EBV, Burkitt's lymphoma, etc. will be given in Chapter 15.

Radiation cancer

If we are to support the view that malignant disease in man results in general from sequential somatic mutation intrinsically determined, the cancer-producing effect of radiation must obviously become a crucial area for discussion. In considering the mutagenic aspects of radiation in an earlier chapter it was impossible to avoid some reference to malignant disease. Both at technical–medical and popular levels the twin dangers of atomic radiation in less than acutely lethal doses are genetic malformations and metabolic defects, on the one hand, and cancer or leukaemia, on the other. Some of the former discussion on ultraviolet and ionizing radiations will have to be traversed again, but this time with all the emphasis on the induction of cancer.

Ultraviolet light has a well defined action in damaging DNA by the production of thymine dimers. There is an equally well understood and effective repair mechanism by which the affected nucleotides are excised and repaired. In persons with little skin pigmentation, and even more so in albinos, prolonged exposure to strong sunlight must give rise to continuing and widespread damage to the DNA of epidermal cells and melanocytes, but for the greater part this is rapidly and effectively repaired. Over the years, however, the incidence of malignancies involving the two types of cell increases: basal cell carcinomas and squamous cell epitheliomas from epidermal cells, malignant melanomas from melanocytes. The high incidence of these tumours in Australia leaves no doubt whatever that exposure to the shorter wavelengths of sunlight and the low level of European pigmentation are both directly concerned in their prevalence.

Another sunlight-induced lesion that has apparently never been studied as closely as it deserves is the ordinary freckling of childhood. The circular shape, distribution and persistence of freckles can most simply be interpreted as resulting from somatic mutation of a type which combines more pigment production per cell and a limited proliferative advantage over unmutated melanocytes. A related phenomenon is seen in albinos of Melanesian or other dark-skinned peoples, who in adolescence develop pigmented spots and patches on skin exposed to sunlight. In all these conditions we have the same options of either placing the whole responsibility on the radiation or seeing the effects as due to the errors introduced in repairing vast numbers of DNA lesions—in other words, a manifestation of intrinsic mutagenesis made possible by the exceptional call for frequent DNA repair.

The origin of skin malignancies associated with exposure to sunlight is strongly correlated with age and, compared with the numbers of cells damaged by ultraviolet radiation, malignancy is extremely rare. There is direct evidence that a gross genetic deficiency in the DNA repair enzymes greatly increases the incidence of cancer in exposed skin, and to that extent supports the concept of intrinsic mutagenesis. Xeroderma pigmentosum is a rare genetic disease of man where the skin is extremely susceptible to exposure to sunlight (or artificial ultraviolet light), with the appearance of excess pigmentation and an exceptionally high incidence of malignancy, both epithelioma and melanoma. The study of cell cultures from such patients[111, 112] has shown that the biochemical defect is an inability to deal with the characteristic thymine dimer lesions owing to the absence or functional weakness of the first (incising) endonuclease of the DNA repair system of enzymes.

Ionizing radiation is well known for its capacity to induce cancer, including leukaemia, in part from the experience of Hiroshima and

Nagasaki, but also from the tragic experience of dial painters using radium- or mesorthorium-based luminous paint in the 1920s, and from the therapeutic use of large doses of X-rays, particularly for ankylosing spondylitis[17]. All effects of ionizing radiation on living cells or tissues are ascribed directly or indirectly to the absorption of energy and the formation of ion pairs (ionization) within the tissues. Very large doses can, of course, be rapidly lethal, but from the medical angle we are concerned only with genetic changes initiated in single cells. Whatever interpretation is placed on the production of cancer or leukaemia by ionizing radiation malignant disease must be accepted as a very rare result of massive numbers of intracellular ionizations. Just as has been found for mutagenicity in the strict sense, the yield of tumours in irradiated animals depends on the period over which a dose of X-rays or γ-rays is applied, as well as the size of the dose. Irradiation at high dose rate is more effective than at a lower rate, indicating that repair of DNA plays a part. The effect is hardly visible with neutron or other types of radiation giving a more intense burst of ionization[113].

There is no evidence that cancer or leukaemia can be induced in any tissue receiving a dose of less than some hundreds of R except for the indirect but impressive evidence that exposure of the pregnant uterus to diagnostic X-rays increases the likelihood of leukaemia and other childhood malignancies in the child subsequently born.

Confining ourselves for the present to post-natal exposure to therapeutic X-rays, there is an approximate indication of a proportionality between dose and biological effect, and, as was indicated in the earlier discussion of mutagenic effects, the convention has been developed of accepting a linear dose–effect (LDE) relationship over the whole range of doses. We can recall that in round figures exposure to a dose of 100 R is taken as producing approximately one case of leukaemia per year per 10 000 people exposed; for 1 R the incidence is one case per million, and correspondingly for even smaller doses.

A brief account taken from the BEIR report[19], and using their conclusions without specific reference to primary sources, may be used to select findings that are relevant to the present discussion. The first point is the selective effect of radiation in favouring the induction of one type of malignancy rather than another. In the Hiroshima–Nagasaki studies, leukaemia cases reaching a peak incidence at seven years after the bombings were more conspicuous than any other, with an absolute risk value for adults of $4.7/10^6/\mathrm{yr}/\mathrm{R}$. Breast and lung showed a value around 1, while stomach and skin cancer showed no evidence of increase.

Both in the atomic bomb studies and in the English work on patients irradiated for spondylitis the leukaemias were acute or chronic myelogenous, with no increase in chronic lymphatic. Table 4 gives a simplified extract of the BEIR report tables, which, having regard to the gross uncertainties in all calculations, probably conveys a legitimate general picture of the situation.

Table 4 Estimates of risk of neoplastic disease from ionizing radiation

Disease	*Ages*	*Absolute risk**	*Relative risk†*
Leukaemia	0–9	2.0	5.0
	10+	1.0	2.0
All other cancers	0–9	1.0	2.0
	10+	5.0	0.2
including:			
Breast ca.	10+	1.5	—
Lung ca.	10+	1.3	—
G-I ca.	10+	1.0	—
Bone ca.	10+	0.2	—
rest	10+	1.0	—

*Absolute risk = deaths per million per R per year; †Relative risk = percentage increase over the spontaneous rate per R (Data from BEIR report[19], p. 171, by courtesy of U.S. Government Printing Office.)

A similarly simplified table may be useful in showing the very small effect that background radiation would have if the LDE rule held and the calculated risk estimates were used to derive the total number of cases that could be due to background (0.1 R per annum) in the United States. As was evident in regard to mutations, the 'spontaneous' occurrence of leukaemia and cancer is so high that it is impossible to recognize the effect, if any, of background or any additional radiation of the same order of magnitude. In the words of the report: 'It is unlikely that the

Table 5 Deaths from leukaemia and cancer in the United States

	Leukaemia	*All other cancers*
Deaths (1967)	14 336	296 647
Calculated effect of background: deaths per annum	738 (5.2%)	2 436 (0.82%)

(Data from BEIR report[19], by courtesy of U.S. Government Printing Office.)

presence or absence of a true threshold for cancer in human populations can be proved.' The same holds for experimental studies, of which one of the most elaborate was that of Finkel *et al*[114]. It is illuminating that their results have been interpreted as favouring a threshold, an LDE relation, and an effect related to the square of the dose by different commentators.

Another feature of special importance to our concentration on age-associated aspects of cancer is the fact that the effect of radiation increases with age approximately parallel to the spontaneous incidence[115]. Although a variety of explanations might be suggested for this, it becomes very difficult to fit with the assumption that the initiating malignant lesion is produced directly by a single radiation episode.

One must also bear in mind the possibility that much of the effect of radiation is not on the DNA of the cell that initiates a tumour, but is much more indirect. The general opinion about X-ray epithelioma of the skin is that it is produced only by very large doses and may be almost wholly associated with radio-dermatitis. This would mean that here the radiation is acting as a co-carcinogen rather than an inducing carcinogen. Salaman and Roe[116], discussing the 'promotion' of tumours, put main stress on hyperplasia, considering that 'hyperplasia is probably necessary for tumour promotion but may not be sufficient'. In view of the known ability of X-rays to break a DNA segment, the minimal effect on human skin may be related to the high efficiency of repair mechanisms for both ultraviolet and X-ray damage to the DNA of epidermal epithelium and melanocytes.

The same conclusion can be drawn for the induction of cancer by radiation as was reached for its mutagenic capacity. The 'spontaneous' development of leukaemia and all the other forms of cancer is far beyond what could be produced by naturally present radiation. The possibility that intrinsic mutagenesis is responsible for most, and perhaps in a special sense for all, malignant disease remains open.

The production of leukaemia by diagnostic irradiation of the foetus during pregnancy

The evidence that leukaemia and other malignant diseases are increased in incidence by exposure to diagnostic X-rays in utero is due mainly to Alice Stewart and her collaborators[117]. Their figures were obtained by comparing the history of X-rays during their foetal life of 6347 children dying from malignant disease under the age of ten between 1953 and

1965 in England and Wales. About 80 per cent of the total deaths were investigated over those thirteen years. An equal number of healthy children chosen as statistically satisfactory controls were also investigated similarly. All the childhood cancers and leukaemia gave approximately similar figures, and, in round figures, 15 per cent of the children with malignant disease and 10 per cent of the control children had been radiated during foetal life. A rough calculation indicates that full coverage would have found 8000 cases from the 8 million children born during the thirteen years.

Of these 8 million, 800 000 were irradiated, with 1200 cases of malignancy, while 7 200 000 were not irradiated, with 6800 cases—rates of $1500/10^6$ and $940/10^6$ respectively, i.e. an excess of $560/10^6$. The average dose to the bone marrow of the foetus could be only roughly estimated, but one can take Stewart's figure for the excess deaths as $572/10^6/R$.

If one uses the LDE rule to calculate how many cases should be produced by background radiation for nine months (0.075 R), acting similarly, the number is approximately $43/10^6$, i.e. less than 1/20 of the actual number, which was $940/10^6$.

Although there has been a good deal of scepticism about retrospective studies of this sort, there has been some confirmatory work[118], and at the present time one judges that the results are accepted as broadly correct.

From our present point of view it is significant that even with the much greater apparent susceptibility which, allowing for the mean time of death from malignancy being about three years, was $190/10^6/R/yr$ as compared with the adult $1/10^6/R/yr$, there are many more spontaneous cases than would be calculated by the LDE rule to be due to background radiation.

The interpretation of antenatally induced malignancy would therefore require no major modification of the hypothesis of intrinsic mutagenesis. Spontaneous error on very rare occasions can be expected to initiate malignant change in foetal cells as elsewhere; the high rate of mitosis and active synthesis may actually make them more prone to error than cells of the adult. In addition, changes distorting growth control are more likely to have a significant effect than in post-natal life. Finally, and perhaps most importantly, any nidus of malignant change in the foetus will not be subject to immune surveillance until some time after birth. Further damage by low dose radiation will increase the need for repair, and hence the likelihood of error. A striking feature of Stewart's figures is that the ratios of percentage irradiated in comparison with normal children did not vary significantly from 15:10 for any of the types of childhood cancer. The only fully established example of human cancer induced in utero by a chemical carcinogen is the vaginal carcinoma seen in young women whose mothers had been treated with diethyl stilboestrol during the relevant pregnancy(119). This could be another example of the high susceptibility of the foetal tissues to mutational change. Extensive recent work(120) has shown a high susceptibility of rat foetuses to the carcinogenic effect of nitrosamines and other conventional carcinogens given intravenously to the pregnant animal.

Chemical carcinogenesis

If neither cancer viruses or natural radiation can be responsible for more than a tiny part of human cancer, it is necessary to look at chemical carcinogens present in the natural environment as the final possibility of an extrinsic cause.

It is inevitable that cancer research, using experimental animals, should concentrate on the study of situations where malignant disease can be produced in a high proportion of individuals in a conveniently short time, usually a quarter or less of the species' lifespan. The effective study of chemical carcinogenesis began with the reproduction of something equivalent to human tar cancer on the ears of rabbits. This led, naturally, to the chemical isolation of the first pure carcinogen, a synthetic polycyclic hydrocarbon of the general type found in tar. A year or two later, one of the major carcinogens of tar was isolated as 3, 4-menzopyrene and shown to be active in tests on mouse skin. Standard methods of demonstrating carcinogenicity in relatively short periods were developed and large numbers of polycyclic hydrocarbons were synthesized and tested. As far as can be judged from a review by Boyland(121), after thirty years' work no satisfactory statement could be made as to how the active types influenced the cell or why the inactive forms did not. Boyland concluded that the target material might be nucleic acid or protein, or even some other type of molecule.

Simultaneously, very large numbers of almost every available type of synthetic organic chemicals were tested, sometimes with hints from industrial experience, more often as simple exploratory experiments. The major groups of alkylating agents, lactones, nitroso compounds and aromatic amines all produced proportions of highly active carcinogens, and a number of new experimental approaches were developed. New types of experimental cancer, notably hepatomas, and fibrosarcomas resulting from intramuscular injection of the carcinogen became standard. Again, judging from a series of reviews in 1964[122], none allowed any clear understanding of the process by which they could induce cancer. During the last decade most laboratory activity has switched away from such work to virological, immunological and genetic fields. Suitable chemical carcinogens are widely used for the initiation of cancer cell lines, but their mode of action has only recently again become an active research topic.

Ames and his collaborators[123, 124] has been interested in developing highly sensitive bacterial mutants as indicators of mutagenic action. They work with a histidine-requiring Salmonella mutant and measure the yield of revertants on appropriate plates. The most sensitive indicator strain is extremely 'rough', without a lipopolysaccharide coat to inhibit entry of carcinogens, is a mutant lacking excision repair activity, and has a 'hot spot' in the relevant locus with the repetitive sequence ... XCGCGCGCGX ... specially suitable for frame shift mutations. Parenthetically, that recital is a striking indirect testimony to the need for and effectiveness of the precautions against potential mutagens that are built into every natural organism. Using such indicator strains, Ames *et al.* could demonstrate frame shift mutagenesis by all of eighteen known carcinogens, provided an activating system, rat liver extract, was added to the test plates. They included such well known agents as methylcholanthrene, benzo(a)pyrene, and aflatoxin B1. The use of the liver extract was based on the work of Miller and Miller[125] on the induction of experimental liver cancer, where the actual inducer is usually a metabolite of the carcinogen administered.

It is of interest to note that with most sensitive indicator the number of revertants per plate from some 2×10^8 bacteria averaged 36 with a range from 21 to 53, while significantly increased numbers after carcinogen addition ranged from 85 to 13 600. The two points to be emphasized are, first, the consistency of the level of spontaneous mutation, and second, that even the highest yield of revertants involved less than one ten-thousandth of the specially sensitive bacteria exposed to the carcinogen. It is only to underline the obvious and the inevitable to reiterate that there are stochastic regularities in biological materials even for happenings whose probability lies between 10^{-5} and 10^{-7}. Degrees of fidelity are measurable even at this level.

The claim that these experiments establish that chemical carcinogens are such in virtue of their power to increase the proportion of mutations can be accepted, as can the adoption of the interpretation by Streisinger *et al.*[126] of the mechanism of frame shift mutation, viz. that the planar molecules of these aromatic compounds can stabilize a mispairing of two bases sufficiently to allow subsequent replication to produce a DNA segment with one base pair in excess or deficient at that point. Either will result in a frame-shift mutation. An important part of the Streisinger interpretation is that the action of the planar molecule is essentially to interfere with the effective repair of a spontaneous fault which otherwise would be rapidly returned to normal.

Most of the actively studied carcinogens have only the slightest possible bearing on human cancer except for a few specific examples that may involve small numbers of people in industry. For our immediate interest in the possible extrinsic origin of the common human cancers we must necessarily confine ourselves to the carcinogens known or reasonably suspected to be present in the general human environment and taken into the body in food, water or air. In a recent review, Roe[20] and Grosso[127] reported on the presence in normal foods of polycyclic hydrocarbons related to benzopyrene, nitrosamines and aflatoxin, but only in extremely minute quantities. Measured in parts per billion (10^9), the amounts were: aflatoxin 110, polycyclic hydrocarbons 50, and nitrosamines 14. In other words, minute traces of mould and bacterial metabolites and of tarry materials inevitably find their way into food.

For what seem to be emotional rather than logical grounds, the same fear is widely held that any carcinogen may show a linear dose–effect relationship down to the smallest amount. If 1 per cent of aflatoxin in food produces liver cancer in one person in a hundred, then 1 part in 10^9 will result in one case per billion people. This view has effectively been included in the law of the United States with the 'Delaney cancer clause' in the 1958 amendment of the Food, Drugs and Cosmetic Act, which specifically excludes the use in foodstuffs of even the smallest amount of any substance which in even the largest possible dose has produced cancer in any experimental animal. Reports of a recent discussion in New York indicate that there is wide support amongst the more vocal scientists for maintaining the Delaney rule.

For a variety of reasons I would consider the attitude quite ridiculous, and not less so the reported opinion of the FDA, that 3×10^6 mice might be the optimal number to use for a definitive test of a suspect material. Roe[20] notes the danger of *any* substance given subcutaneously in mice or rats producing inflammatory fibrosarcomas. Anyone aware of the human problems of maintaining a few thousand, let alone a few million, mice free from infection and from a variety of recognized and unrecognized accidents for the whole of life would unhesitatingly condemn the 'megamouse' experiments as illusory and liable to be seriously misleading.

The fear that some of the hundreds of chemicals that deliberately or by accident are added to food or in some other way are taken into the body may be responsible for cancer is almost certainly groundless. Apart from an apparent increase in leukaemia, which is probably due to better diagnosis of leukaemia as a cause of death, and which has ceased since 1970[128], and the massive rise in lung cancer, there has been no significant

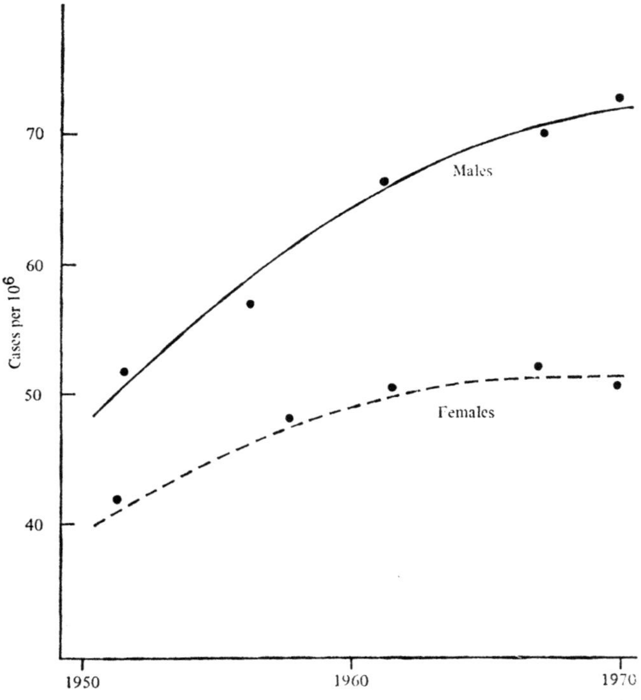

Figure 14 To show the incidence of deaths from leukaemia (all forms) in Australia. As in other countries, the rise has virtually ceased by 1970 in males, while the female rate has been nearly stable since 1955

increase in any of the major forms of cancer since the beginning of the century. Exposure of very large numbers of people to DDT for over thirty years, and of the whole world's population for nearly twenty years, has shown none of the increase in liver cancer that was once feared. Only in the very special circumstance of highly radioactive elements, such as radium in bone, do trace amounts to anything cause cancer. Even here the equivalent R dosage needed to produce bone sarcoma in 50 per cent of those subject to industrial exposure was very large in terms of normal background radiation or diagnostic X-rays.

The reader can probably sense the direction in which this discussion is leading. Despite about seventy years' intensive scientific work aimed at identifying a cause or a series of causes of human cancer, the only demographically significant success has been to establish that polycyclic hydrocarbons taken into the body in cigarette smoking or by various forms of industrial exposure can cause cancer from prolonged and extensive action. A number of industrial examples of cancer induction by other types of material are known, but involve very small numbers of people. Many other chemical and viral agents have been suggested, but for the present the evidence for their importance involves only animals other than man.

Biological place of cancer

If radiations, non-biological chemicals, some products of bacterial and fungal metabolism, and viruses are responsible only for a few well defined types of malignant disease, and in the case of the first three agents only after intense and prolonged exposure, we are left with the great mass of malignant disease unaccounted for on any straightforward cause–effect relationship. After nearly twenty years' intense interest in what I have tended to call a Darwinian approach to the behaviour of clonally proliferating cells in the body, it was inevitable that I should want to expand the approach which has been relatively successful in its application, as the concept of clonal selection, to immunological theory and bring something of the same attitude to malignant disease. Before 1957, all approaches towards explaining the obvious relationship between the injection of an antigen into a rabbit and the production of a corresponding antibody a week later required the antigen (or part of it) to provide a template from which the information needed to produce a specific antibody was derived. In fact the antibody patterns arise by intrinsic genetic processes producing a diversity of random patterns from which circumstances, pre-eminently the presence of antigen, select certain types for production. The analogous approach to malignant disease is to assume that the basic changes in somatic cell DNA, which result in the cell taking on the overt neoplastic character, are of intrinsic genetic origin and related in some way to evolutionary needs; and that during the period of youth and maturity there are effective means of preventing such genetic changes producing harmful manifestations.

The basis for a primary interpretation of cancer in terms of an intrinsic genetic origin is contained in the general theory of ageing that was outlined in the preceding chapter. In its application to cancer the first requirement is to establish as clearly as possible that the development of a malignant clone results from one or more somatic mutations as defined earlier. There stress was laid on the importance of monoclonality in indicating that a tumour or other pathological condition had arisen by the clonal proliferation of a single cell and *ipso facto* had arisen by somatic mutation or some equivalent process. Fialkov[129] has recently reviewed the findings obtained by the study of tumours in women or female children who were heterozygous for variants of the G6PD enzyme. Since most solid tumours contain varying amounts of non-malignant tissues which will inevitably show evidence of both variants, it is important to test pieces of tumour tissue as free as possible from non-malignant cells and be prepared to find a certain amount of 'noise' in the results. It is perhaps of special interest that four tumour types derived from cells of the lymphocyte–immunocyte series were uniformly monoclonal in Fialkov's hands. They were, first, Burkitt's lymphoma, a tumour predominantly of African children, which has a unique restriction to heavily malarious regions of central Africa and is discussed at some length in Chapter 15; the others were lymphosarcoma (five instances), reticulum cell sarcoma (two), and plasmacytoma (three). The monoclonality of the last named can be even more impressively demonstrated by the homogeneity of the immunoglobulin (myeloma protein) produced by the cells. Carcinomas of skin and mucous surfaces given only a relatively small proportion of indubitably monoclonal tumours, but a variable proportion showing both types of enzyme may be false results owing to an unsuspected high proportion of non-malignant stroma and infiltrating cells. Single examples of monoclonal melanoma and neuroblastoma are on record, and most ovarian teratomata, which, being derivatives of the germ cells, can sometimes show monoclonality by tests with enzymes controlled by autosomal genes, are definitely monoclonal.

The only outstandingly non-monoclonal malingnant condition is multiple neurofibromatosis. Here the condition is an inherited one, and one assumes a high likelihood of unrelated somatic mutation providing a second necessary event relatively late in development. Although it has not to my knowledge been tested for monoclonality, special mention should be made of another tumour in which both germ-line and somatic mutations may be concerned. Retinoblastoma is a tumour of early childhood involving only immature retinoblasts in the eye and therefore never arising after the first year of life. It is one of the few specific types of human tumour that have a well established genetic basis. Surgical treatment is often effective and enough family histories are available to characterize the inheritance as of a dominant gene. The inheritance is not, however, invariably demonstrable, and according to Knudson[(130)], who has analysed the family history of large numbers of cases, both germ-line and somatic mutations are involved. In his view, for a tumour to arise, two sequential mutations from normal, A and B, are required. B is always somatic, but for it to induce the tumour the cell concerned must already carry the mutant gene A. This may have been inherited as a germ-line anomaly from an ancestral mutation or it, too, may have arisen as a primary somatic mutation. A large proportion of infants with retinoblastomas show more than one tumour; these are all individuals with A as a germ-line quality. Those in whom two sequential somatic mutations are responsible will always show only a single tumour. From his data and a fairly complex chain of biological and mathematical reasoning Knudson concluded that the frequency of mutation A in a germ-line cell was approximately equal to the rate of its appearance as a primary somatic mutation in retinoblasts. In a more recent paper, Knudson and Strong[(108)] found that two other tumours of not very dissimilar character could be treated similarly. Neuroblastoma gave results very similar to retinoblastoma. Phaeochromocytoma appears later in life than the other two, but with appropriate adjustment also conformed to the sequential mutation model.

There are almost certainly less conspicuous examples of genetic influence on the readiness with which malignant disease emerges. In general, however, one must accept Doll's[(39)] conclusion that the characteristic increase of cancer incidence with age, according to a 'power law', calls as a minimum for a multistage mechanism of two or more steps, each an independent mutational event and each providing some selective advantage to the mutant clone.

Once such a point of view has been accepted, one can make the basic assumption that, for steps in the induction of malignancy, the same rules hold as for any other type of cumulative somatic mutation. The error in DNA duplication, recombination or repair is related to the structure of the DNA-polymerase or other key enzymes concerned; the effect of damage by intrusion of physical, chemical or viral agents is to increase the opportunities for error by enzymes in the course of attempted repair. By hypothesis the biological function of this infidelity in replication is to allow expression of the characteristic lifespan of the species. Obviously the time available to an animal before the degenerations of senescence set in is an important facet of the life style of the species and an appropriate value is an evolutionary necessity. Some way of achieving it must be found within the limitations of the evolutionary process, and if the effective way of achieving it has side effects, which may be disastrous to individuals but have no evolutionary relevance, this will not detract in the least from its effectiveness or its persistence. One of those side effects, we believe, is cancer.

Here I should like to make a short diversion to a somewhat analogous situation, the sickle cell gene in Africa. This is a mutant gene which modifies the structure of the haemoglobin molecule so that it disturbs the function of the red cells of the blood, particularly when the gene is in double dose. Heterozygotes with only one abnormal gene can be recognized as carriers of the so called sickle cell trait, but show no more than trivial evidence of any ill effect. Under some circumstances the heterozygous condition is positively beneficial in making such people better able to resist chronic malaria, an advantage that is presumably responsible for the existence of 10 per cent or more people with the gene in malarious regions of Africa. If among a hundred heterozygotes an additional five individuals survived because of this advantage, this would more than counterbalance the 0.25 per cent of all births that were homozygous for the gene.

In pre-colonial days the infantile mortality among Africans was probably of the order of 10–30 per cent, and any children born with sickle cell anaemia would undoubtedly have died in infancy. If we use 10 per cent as the probable proportion of heterozygotes and assume that these have a 5 per cent better chance of surviving childhood malaria than normal children, a rough calculation of the advantage can be made. In a population of 1000 with 100 heterozygous individuals and the rest normals, the proportion of marriages involving two heterozygotes would be 1 per cent, and in the families of these, one child in four would be homozygous and die from sickle cell anaemia. Where heterozygote marries normal, 50 per cent of the children are heterozygotes. To obtain a stabilized situation, only a 0.25 per cent advantage to the heterozygote is necessary. If the advantage is more than that, the percentage of heterozygotes in the population will rise. At the 10 per cent level the deaths of a fraction of 1 per cent of children would be quite unnoticed and biologically tolerable. Nature has no concern with what is unimportant for evolution, whether this is death in early life from a harmful double recessive trait or death after the reproductive period from cancer.

A somatic mutational origin of malignant disease has been frequently postulated over many years and in most respects the interpretation I have adopted corresponds fairly closely with the approach used by Burch in his 1965 papers[131, 132]. In these, his summaries include the following points: Each stage of the initiation represents some form of somatic mutation, probably of nuclear genes. Some subpopulations have a genetically based predisposition to a particular type of malignancy. In regard to leukaemia, the germ cell mutational frequency is approximately the same as that applicable to somatic cells over the whole lifespan. Early leukaemia requires one inherited mutation and two somatic mutations: a condition of stress (which may be viral) is then necessary for malignant development.

The only novelty in the present approach is an attempt to provide a basis for the characteristic rate of somatic mutation which must be postulated to exist in any theory that can account for the quantitive character of the age-association of cancer. If the somatic mutations that are responsible in one way and another for the primary and secondary attributes of senescence have the same basic source as those which lead to overt malignancy, it is reasonable enough to expect both to show a similar pattern of development with age. It would not be proper, however, to attempt a more comprehensive discussion of the point until the equally, or perhaps more, important influence of immune surveillance is discussed.

CHAPTER 13

MALIGNANT DISEASE—2

In many ways cancer is as complex and ill defined a concept as old age itself. Probably no two tumours ever show the same clinical and histological pattern, and there is enough on record to make one equally confident that adequate biochemical (especially enzymological), immunological and ultrastructural study of tumour cells in culture would show an equal diversity. The one great regularity to be observed in cancer is the consistency of its age-specific incidence curve, with its typical association in all species with the period of senescence. It is almost solely with this association that I am concerned, but, if it is to be understood, the other general aspects of malignant disease must be looked at in sequence.

Cellular aspects of carcinogenesis

The essence of a malignant tumour is the relative, sometimes almost absolute, autonomy of its cells. Experimentally, a tumour can be defined by the capacity of its cells to proliferate when transferred in relatively small numbers to the tissues of a syngeneic host, and, subject to borderline qualifications inevitable in any attempt at biological generalization, this differentiates malignant from normal cells. The crux of the problem is to define the various differences that distinguish a malignant cell from normal cells of the same lineage.

As I have discussed earlier, the basic difference is 'somatic genetic' in the sense that the special qualities of the cancer cell are transmissible to all descendant cells. Yet it would be completely inadequate to ascribe the overt appearance of cancer simply to mutational changes. There are so many examples of environmental agents and intrinsic factors, such as hormone levels, having an influence on the incidence of cancer that the final clinical expression must be dependent not only on multistage mutation but also on many non-genetic factors. There are for instance, as I have mentioned earlier, several types of cancer which may show a clear genetic component in the ordinary sense, such as retinoblastoma and phaeochromocytoma. In each, however, an additional somatic mutation is necessary. There are well established premalignant conditions, both in clinical experience and experimental work, whose nature is far from being fully understood. Often both somatic mutation and inflammatory conditions may be interacting. Once a tumour is manifest, progressive changes are almost the rule, with the development of increased malignancy and host range, chromosomal abnormalities, and so on.

It is clear that mutation towards cancer must always be against the background of the genetic (i.e. germ-line) potentialities of the cell line involved, and on occasion a mutant gene acquired in some previous generation has a specific role in allowing the appearance of a tumour. Sequential somatic mutation is probably the rule and, as Doll(39) comments, there is little evidence in most cases as to whether two or any number up to seven random episodes are involved. There is an equal absence of information about the extent of proliferative advantage that follows each mutational step. Rather casual evidence from isolated experimental or clinical observations has indicated that premalignant change may be associated with proliferative advantage; and there are other situations in which it seems highly likely that premalignant cells are more or less selectively stimulated by agents which are not in any sense mutagenic. Once a high proliferative advantage is manifested, the opportunity for further sequential mutation increases, and the common production of ectopic products by lung carcinoma and other tumours suggests that mutation *after* malignant change has been established may be of very varied types and is at least not incompatible with the activity of some 'mutator' genes.

For many years oncologists have looked to changes in cell surface structure for an interpretation of the loss of morphostatic control, which is the primary characteristic of a tumour. A recent hypothesis due to Holley(133) puts a different slant to the significance of membrane changes. In his view, normal cell growth in the body, although influenced by many other factors, is proximately determined by the concentration inside the cell of one or more low molecular weight nutrients. Their entry is controlled by transport mechanisms in the cell surface which, according to need or on hormonal stimulation, allow selective passage of the components needed from the standard circulating mixture. Cancer could be associated with a wide variety of somatic genetic lesions involving, for example, changes in the amount or activity of a transport protein, or in cell membrane structure, modification of cyclic AMP metabolism, a change in availability or affinity of hormone receptor sites, and so on.

Once a suitable mutation or combination of mutations has given rise to an active tumour growing by virtue of some distortion of the membrane transport mechanism, a classical Darwinian situation has been instituted. There may be frequent further mutations, but all mutants not capable of effective competition will be rapidly eliminated and only 'progressive' mutants of higher malignancy will overgrow the existing cell population.

One of the major weaknesses of genetic theory is in regard to the function, control and scope for mutational change in the components of the somatic cell genome other than structural genes. Every nucleus seems to contain much more DNA than can be ascribed to structural genes, and it is to be presumed that non-structural functions are active in malignant cells and highly likely to present some functional distortions associated with malignancy.

Of well defined cellular phenomena, perhaps the type most likely to depend on non-structural genes is the occurrence of a switch from production and use of one protein to an alternative, at some point in differentiation or in response to some physiological requirement. Two well known examples are the successive changes in haemoglobin from embryonic to foetal to adult, corresponding to the sequence of δ, γ, β in one pair of chains; and the switch of an immunocyte to produce successively monomeric IgM, IgM, IgG. The fact that many, perhaps most, malignant cells produce foetal antigens, while it is common for protein hormones or other ectopic proteins to be produced in fully developed clinical cancers, indicates that changes of the same sort can go on after malignant change and, probably by implication, at intermediate stages before the change is complete. One suspects that as soon as better means of defining and recognizing non-structural mutation are available there will be a flush of hypotheses about its bearing on malignant disease.

It is impossible to say whether non-structural genes are involved in any of the environmental effects on the development of overt malignancy. It is a possibility, but it seems wiser to look for effects that do not involve DNA at all.

Environmental (promotional) effects

Berenblum[134, 134a] showed many years ago that treatment of mice for a brief period with a carcinogenic hydrocarbon might have no capacity to produce a skin carcinoma unless the treated area were subsequently treated with an irritant, croton resin, in the first experiments, which had no demonstrable carcinogenic effect alone. The potentiality to respond to the co-carcinogen could persist for a year or more. One can find a wide variety of more or less analogous findings. Trauma and repair may acts as a co-carcinogen to a site prepared, as in Berenblum's experiments. In another context (see page 000) I mention Curtis's finding[52], that mice given a substantial dose of whole body X-irradiation become susceptible to developing hepatomas when regeneration occurs after carbon tetrachloride necrosis. Smithers[135] speaks of the common clinical experience of seeing neoplasia develop at the edge of a chronic ulcer. Breast cancer is often a slow development from precancerous change and can sometimes be demonstrated to be of multi-centric origin. Here, too, inflammatory and reparative changes have probably been at work.

The development of malignancy in cell cultures of 'fibroblasts' from normal mouse tissues is relevant in relation to these *in vivo* experiences. According to Franks[136], 30 or 40 per cent of such cultures, after repeated passage for nine months, produce tumours when injected into syngeneic animals. The proportion was not significantly different when the cultures were started with cells from foetal, young or aged mice. Workers in Heidelberger's laboratory[137] used cells from the ventral prostate of C3H mice. As the cells were aneuploid, they cannot be regarded as wholly normal; nevertheless the primary organ cultures never produced tumours. When methylcholanthrene (MCA), a potent carcinogen, was added to plates seeded with ± 1000 cells from a primary culture, a proportion of the plates showed the development of one or a small number of heaped up areas with the characteristic appearance of a colony of transformed cells. Such changed cells, but not the single-layered background cells, produced tumours when injected into syngeneic mice. Since only one or two cells per thousand responded in this fashion, one of the possibilities is that these cells were precancerous mutants stimulated to rapid growth by the MCA and taking on malignant quality by the appearance of a secondary mutant in the population that resulted. The alternative favoured by the authors would be that in something less than 1 per cent of the normal cells the action of the MCA produced a mutation, allowing full development of malignancy. A decision between the two possibilities could be made by quantitative testing of the transformed cell colonies for tumour-producing power at various stages of growth. Since each of the tumours that could be tested immunologically carried an individual tumour-specific antigen, the second hypothesis requires the simultaneous occurrence at a frequency about 10^{-3} of two unrelated mutations in a single cell. This is probably in itself enough to prove that any effect of the MCA was not that of a mutagen. A third possibility would assume that in the primary cell culture there were small numbers of cells with full malignant potentiality but requiring some mitotic stimulus to induce proliferation. Once proliferation had begun, it would be assumed to continue; there are precedents from cell culture experiments which allow one to picture the production of mitotic stimulants by proliferating cells, so providing an automatic goad to continuing proliferation.

One can summarize this discussion as a recognition of the complexity of normal cellular controls and an attempt to work out the implications for cancer of the hypothesis that most somatic mutations are of intrinsic origin and derived from the quota of errors inherent in the structure of the enzymes concerned with monitoring, replication and repair of DNA. It has been assumed throughout that the classical chemical carcinogens do not act directly as mutagens in the sense that they or a metabolite react with DNA to change the genome into one characteristic of a malignant mutant cell. The assumption is that damage to DNA is either such as to render any descendant cell non-viable or to call for the necessary repair process, mutation being the manifestation of some relatively minor inaccuracy in the repair process that still leaves a viable gene. A related suggestion has recently been made in a review by Haddow[(138)], where he asks 'whether carcinogens produce by direct chemical action an enzymatic defect of the same general character as is produced in xeroderma pigmentosum by purely genetic means'. It will be recognized that Haddow's suggestion still calls for an 'instructive' process differing categorically from the stochastic character of intrinsic mutagenesis.

Almost every other worker in the field, however, still assumes automatically that the impact of a carcinogen is directly mutagenic by its chemical action on the DNA of the cell that gives rise to the transformed clone. Doll[(39)], for instance, summarizes his approach to the age incidence of cancer by formulating the relationship between incidence and age in the equation $I = b(t-w)^k$, where I is the incidence of cancer, t the age of subjects at risk and $(t-w)$ the duration of effective exposure, b is proportional to the mean daily dose of the agent or, better, the mean dose per mitotic cycle, and k is approximately 4.

The work of Ames *et al.*[123, 124] in demonstrating the capacity of many standard carcinogens to produce frame shift mutations in bacteria was described in the preceding chapter, and one may be tempted to think of this as a specific mechanism for creating mutants. It is, however, at least as likely even in bacteria that the emergence of such a mutant depends on repair processes biased towards a frame shift deletion, perhaps by the type of interaction of carcinogen with DNA. The point must never be forgotten that all the processes that intervene between the initial normal cell and the overtly malignant cell must allow the maintenance of full viability and all that this entails. Every random damage must be monitored, recognized, and appropriately repaired if the genome is to remain viable, and this holds even if some types of damage may lead to a higher yield of errors than others.

The environmental influence as exemplified in lung cancer

A majority of writers on the pathology of cancer are concerned still to find environmental causes, and I have touched briefly on some of the factors that have been incriminated. Nevertheless I have put all the emphasis on an intrinsic generation of somatic mutations as the primary source of the whole variety of malignant tumours in man. Cancer has all the hall-marks of an unwanted but inescapable by-product of some process required for a different purpose, and I have speculated that it is related to the means by which the genome determines the appropriate lifespan for the species.

However, the part played by the environmental factors cannot just be swept under the carpet. There is a certain logical untidiness in ascribing most forms of malignant disease to an intrinsic process unrelated to the environment and at the same time accepting cigarette cancer of the lung as of indubitably environmental origin. Most pathologists would consider that the convincing association of cigarette smoking with lung cancer provides a prima facie case for assuming that all epithelial neoplasms result from environmental factors. They will reject the concept of intrinsic mutagenesis as the basic factor in cancer etiology on the grounds that in several instances it is incompatible with the established role of environmental factors and inevitably primary carcinoma of the lung will be at the centre of the discussion.

Help in understanding will naturally be sought from the results of experimental work by Berenblum and his successors on promoting agents. Of the various explanations that have been suggested for these promoting or co-carcinogenic effects, the simplest is that the secondary agent allows an increased selective proliferation of precancerous cells that have already undergone a relevant somatic mutation. This accelerates the accumulation of a large enough population of primary mutants to give a significant likelihood of a second mutation towards malignancy. Clearly, one must leave open the possibility that long exposures to cigarette smoke or other environmental carcinogens may act in similar fashion to allow proliferation of a precancerous, or perhaps sometimes a pre-precancerous, cell or cell line that has arisen by somatic mutation. With progressive enlargement of the preneoplastic clone, the final overtly cancerous mutant will eventually emerge. Another hypothesis that has often been considered would postulate the need for some extrinsic trigger to release a cell already carrying the full genetic character of malignancy from some local constraint.

Some support for both approaches can be found. It is a relatively common occurrence for a tumour to arise in the wound scar many years after a breast has been removed for cancer. The most likely interpretation is that a cancer cell lodged there at the time of operation and was held inert but still viable by the cellular environment that developed. Tumours associated with organs subject to relatively strict hormonal control frequently respond to positive or negative changes in the appropriate hormone levels. Local hormones (chalones) may also be relevant in determining the degree to which malignancy is expressed. The evident high susceptibility of foetal cells to carcinogenesis may be rather directly related to the high level of all types of cellular metabolic activities at the time.

In support of the other suggestion is Brand's work[139, 140] on the induction of tumours by implantation of plastic films in mice. By using two CBA strains differing only by the presence or absence of the marker gene T6, he was able to show that single specific cell clones became firmly attached to the film and on transfer to the opposite mouse type always allowed production of tumour of the donor type. The tumours resulting were quite diverse in character, ranging from highly differentiated fibrosarcoma to an aplastic round cell sarcoma with giant cells. Many showed chromosomal abnormalities. Here there is clearly a possibility that any premalignant cell (of spontaneous origin) finds an opportunity for free proliferation as a single-layered sheet of cells on the plastic surface, an opportunity which would not be available in its absence and which is apparently associated with a capacity to prevent the establishment on the surface of any potentially competitive precancerous clone. Only in this way is the premalignant cell able to build up a large enough clone for a sequential mutation to full malignancy to occur.

At this point another highly relevant problem must be faced: how to adapt a somatic mutational etiology to the wide difference of incidence of cancer in different tissues. Most of the preferred sites have, like the bronchial localization of primary lung cancer, some fairly obvious relationship to environmental irritation and there is an obvious tendency to regard the irritation as the 'cause' of the cancer. Yet such a simple-minded view cannot be an acceptable explanation of the fact that all the commoner types of cancer, with only minor modifications, show the characteristic age-specific incidence that points to sequential mutation as the basic process.

The comonest sites of *fatal* cancer are, in order: lung (predominantly in males), intestine and rectum, stomach, and breast; then follows the group of tumours of lymphocytes and other blood cells, including leukaemia. Two very common but less lethal forms are of skin and cervix uteri. I believe it is reasonable to concentrate on these seven commonest forms to see whether the concept of cancer arising by intrinsic mutagenesis could be a valid one. The group containing what I would call tumours of the immunocyte series, which included Hodgin's disease, lymphosarcoma, reticulum cell sarcoma, chronic lymphatic leukaemia, and multiple myelomatosis, with the more complex conditions of Burkitt's lymphoma and the acute leukaemias of childhood, can be left for discussion in Chapter 15. All the others are tumours of clonally proliferating epithelial cell lines and all are subject to intrinsic or extrinsic stimulation to episodic or continuous physiological proliferation. (1) The bronchial epithelium is damaged and replaced with each episode of influenza and other viral infections; it is subject to inflammatory and proliferative changes by cigarette smoke and other air pollutants and bacteria. (2) The small and large intestines, including the rectum, are lined by proliferating epithelium and are constantly exposed to potentially damaging bacteria and toxic substances passing along the gut as well as to occasional episodes of more specific infection with diarrhoea or dysentery. Epithelial cells are constantly being lost and replaced. The great bulk of intestinal malignancies are in large intestine and rectum. Two factors, one genetic and one environmental, may be significant. Benign polyps are common in the large bowel, multiple polyposis is a well known genetic condition with a strong predisposition to malignancy, and it has been suggested that single lesions may also be genetic in origin. The incidence of cancer of the colon is very much higher in England and America than in Africa; differences in the bacterial flora of the bowel as influenced by the type of food eaten have been suggested as the most likely reason[141]. Tumours in the small intestine are remarkably few, probably because of the very rapid turnover and shedding of the epithelium, which may well get rid of the vast majority of premalignant mutants before they can initiate local proliferation. (3) Stomach cancers are concentrated near the pylorus, where again there is a constantly renewed epithelium regularly subject to minimal or more than minimal traumatization from food. (4) The breast epithelium has its monthly cycle of proliferation and atrophy, as has (5) the cervix uteri, where, in addition, there are the damaging effects of early and frequent intercourse, often asosciated with *Herpes simplex* virus 2 and other low grade infection, as well as the trauma of pregnancy. Finally, (6) the skin epithelium is constantly being renewed, keratinized and lost, and intermittently stimulated to increased proliferation by solar exposure.

There are recognizably similar factors at work in each instance, and it we are concerned to apply the concept of intrinsic mutagenesis to the group it should be sufficient to concentrate on the best known and most important example.

In applying a concept of this sort to the specific instance of cigarette cancer of the lung we must first note the results of histological study of bronchial epithelium in heavy smokers who have died from some cause other than lung cancer. Such autopsies consistently show a variety of proliferative premalignant lesions[142], and there seems to be a real possibility that the essential action of the carcinogen is to provide a situation where cells already modified by mutation can multiply sufficiently to allow the possibility of the additional mutation needed for the full development of malignancy. The effect of this suggestion would be to confine the action of prolonged exposure to cigarette smoke to the terminal stage of the process of intrinsic carcinogenesis. One accepts the straight line character of the specific age-incidence curve as requiring the occurrence of two to five sequential mutations with some proliferative advantage occurring at one or more stages. If the penultimate precancerous cells had a relatively low probability of undergoing the

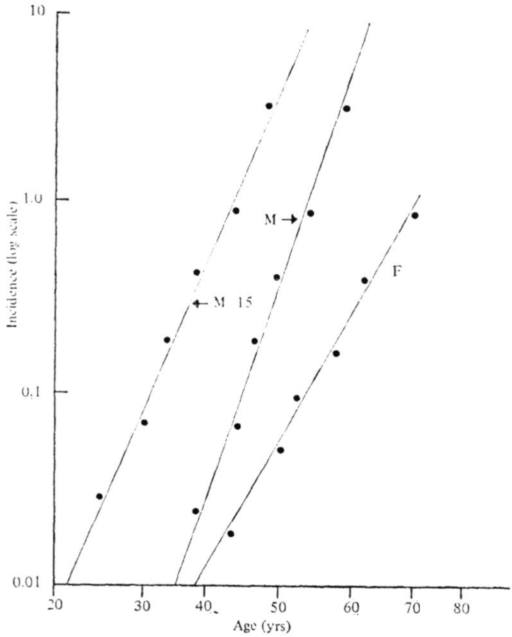

Figure 15 Age incidence of lung cancer deaths in persons born in 1880–1885 in England and Wales. Both age and age-specific incidence are on logarithmic scales. F = female; M = male, with normal age scale; M − 15: males with age fifteen taken as zero to show conversion of the graph to a straight line parallel with the female graph. (From Burnet(143), by courtesy of ***Papua New Guinea med. J.***)

final necessary mutation, their non-malignant proliferation under the complex irritating effect of tobacco smoke constituents would shorten the time required and steepen the curve, probably without change from an approximate straight line. Support for this interpretation can be found in a figure that I have previously published in a different context(143). It shows the age-specific incidence curves for primary lung cancer of male and female cohorts born between 1880–1885 in England and Wales(144). To a reasonable approximation, a large proportion of the males smoked cigarettes by the time of the First World War, when they were thirty, but very few of the women of that cohort would ever have smoked. The female curve can then be taken as respresenting unmodified intrinsic carcinogenesis. The male curve is strikingly steeper. Adopting Doll's view that the important factor is the duration of exposure to the carcinogen and assuming that the males on the average began to smoke at age fifteen, the same values for incidence are plotted with the age at death shown minus 15. It will be seen that the two curves become parallel, as Doll had previously shown with other material.

This is probably the most important justification for Doll's equation $I = b\,(t-w)^k$ previously discussed, but it does not necessarily prove that it is correct. In principle, the matter could be clarified if adequate figures were available of the lung cancer risk in males who had started smoking at fifteen or earlier and in another group beginning after age thirty. Such material is difficult to find, but Doll and Pike[(145)] mention that those *heavy* smokers who start late have a considerably higher level of lung cancer than those starting early. Burch[(146)] quotes a finding of Passey's that an enquiry about the age at which cigarette smoking started among a considerable number of lung cancer patients allowed the collection of two small groups of thirty to forty individuals; one had started before fourteen, the other after thirty. The mean age of both groups was not significantly different (sixty-one years). Both sets of findings indicate that age may be just as important as the intensity and duration of smoking.

I would still feel that the overall results can be equally interpreted as part of a very complex pattern of inflammatory, proliferative and cytolytic processes initiated in bronchial mucosa by which the course of an intrinsically generated sequence of mutational steps is modified. Proliferation of mutant epithelial cells in the precancerous line has been accelerated and the likelihood of later stages arising has been increased at all stages.

Some evidence pointing in the same direction of the importance of age, even in cancers 'obviously' produced by a carncinogen, can be found in quite different fields. Several types of industrial cancer are induced more readily the later exposure begins, and in the studies of leukamia in irradiated spondylitis cases there is a clearly increasing risk with age. The incidence curve with age is essentially parallel to the spontaneous curve from the general population, but about a hundred times the value (Figure 16).

My interpretation, which is quite old-fashioned, is that in all the epithelial cancers I have mentioned we are primarily concerned with intrinsic mutagenesis, always a sequence of two or more mutations being needed and always at random. The chance of a further mutational step towards overt malignancy will always depend on the degree to which the earlier mutant has been able to proliferate. Any extrinsic agent increasing

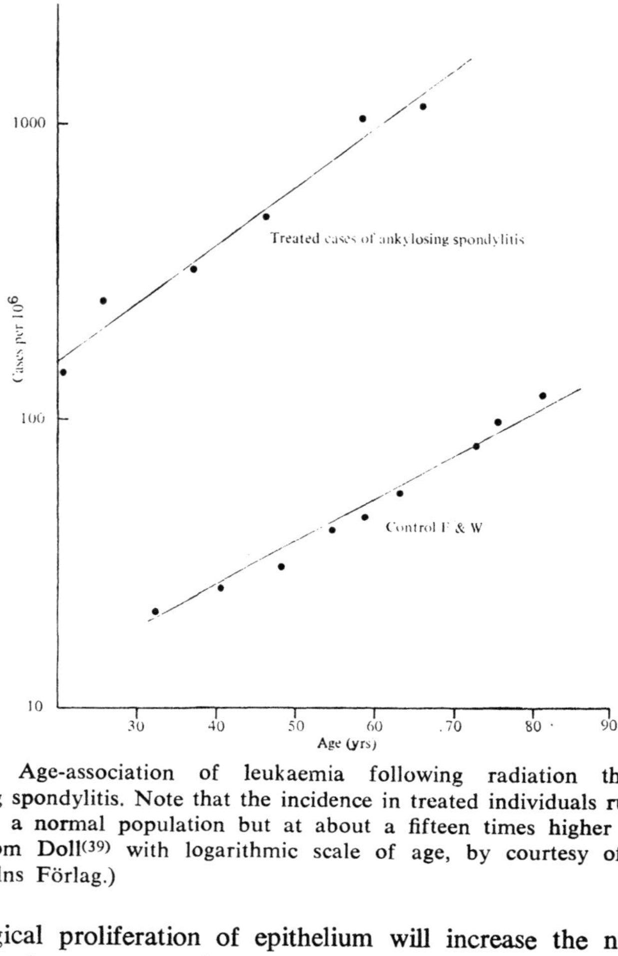

Figure 16 Age-association of leukaemia following radiation therapy for ankylosing spondylitis. Note that the incidence in treated individuals runs parallel to that in a normal population but at about a fifteen times higher level. (Redrawn from Doll[39] with logarithmic scale of age, by courtesy of Nordiska Bokhandelns Förlag.)

physiological proliferation of epithelium will increase the number of candidates for error and, although I have seen no evidence on the point, could be expected to favour selectively the proliferation of premalignant variants over cells not modified in this direction. The sequence to full malignancy will be completed earlier, but it will make use of the same process of sequential mutation.

Conclusion

It is only too evident that where circumstances make a clear-cut experimental decision impossible, any reasonably ingenious theorist can produce a persuasive case for his chosen alternative. There are probably as many pathologists who look for an environmental cause, viral, chemical or physical, for all malignant disease as there were immunologists who believed in Pauling's theory of antibody production in the 1950s. They can produce cogent arguments that some of the chemical carcinogens are so reactive with DNA that the effect must surely be a direct one, and that in experimental virus-induced tumours portion of the viral genome can be identified in the cell DNA.

None of these arguments are decisive; all the observations on which they depend can equally be interpreted as mere secondary effects on intrinsically producd somatic mutations. It is incontestable that minute amounts of alkylating reagents or other reactive material intruding into a nucleus can produce serious structural damage to DNA. Our contention would be that the damage was either irreparable, with subsequent failure of mitosis and death, or of such a degree that repair was possible. With large numbers of cells under repair, as would be the case in any standard experimental test for chemical carcinogenesis, the error-proneness of the enzymes concerned would have a proportionately larger opportunity to be manifested than if only normal mitotic duplication of DNA had been called for.

At the risk of overstating the position, it seems likely that for any type of mutation to be imposed on an otherwise viable cell it must be one that results from specialized activity of a DNA repair or duplicating enzyme. One is reminded of Yanowsky's finding(11) that in the 'mutator' strain of *E. coli* that he worked with all the mutants identified showed that they had resulted from a unidirectional replacement of an A–T pair by G–C. This is in no way comparable to the effect of a crude intrusion into the nucleus by a reactive chemical.

Two other arguments against the direct action of carcinogens on DNA should be kept in mind, although neither seems to have the general validity of the first. Prehn(147) and others have found a well marked immunosuppressive action of several standard carcinogens, including methylcholanthrene. This makes it possible that one additional factor in its effect is to inhibit locally the immune response that in its absence would have eliminated any initiated focus of malignant cells.

Finally, the point made in the previous chapter (see page 133) should be repeated, that on any form of remotely reasonable calculation from the effect of gross doses of radiation the observed incidence of genetic damage and of malignant disease is far greater than could be ascribed to the available environmental agents.

CHAPTER 14

IMMUNE SURVEILLANCE

If it is true that the appearance of malignant cells is a necessary by-product of the mechanism of ageing, there would seem to be a need for some means of countering such accidents, should they occur during the biologically significant years of life from conception to maturity. The most widely held opinion is that partial control is exerted by the immune system and that some of the increased incidence of malignant disease in later life is due to the progressive weakening of this control—the fade-out of immune surveillance[(148)].

This concept has already been touched on in earlier chapters dealing with immunity in relation to ageing. Here we are concerned more directly with the cancer cell as a recognizably foreign object and the degree of effectiveness of immune surveillance in diminishing the incidence of cancer.

Any process by which a nidus of cancer cells recognized as foreign can be removed immunologically must necessarily be similar or identical to what happens when transplanted tissue from another individual of the same species is rejected. The phenomena of homograft rejection have only partial relevance to the theme of cancer control, but it is of considerable interest in relation to the general problem of the development of diversity in genetically determined proteins, enzymes, antigens or antibodies.

The basis of individuality

On several occasions I have considered the implication of the universal finding amongst vertebrates that a tissue graft from one individual to another is invariably rejected unless we are working with identical twins or with specially bred pure-line strains of experimental animal. 'Pure-line strains' are never found in nature, and when we consider the elaborate mechanisms that have developed in forms as far apart as flowering plants and colonial ascidians to prevent self-fertilization, it is clear that there is some very important evolutionary reason for this ban. In nature there can be nothing directly equivalent to the laboratory procedures of skin or organ grafting. Most population geneticists would probably regard the basic reason as the need to foster evolutionary flexibility by always maintaining in the species population a wide diversity of unexpressed genes—of genetic potentiality. Until we can find some basis for understanding the significance of histocompatibility genes and antigens more closely related to the realities of evolution than the artificial findings of the transplantation laboratory, they could still be thought of as mere neutral polymorphisms with no bearing on survival, and therefore wholly adventitious by-products of the more important requirement.

For reasons that may be more intuitive than logical, any immunologist will find that attitude unacceptable and look for some immunologically relevant reason for the universal diversity of histocompatibility antigens. At different times I have suggested three different evolutionary reasons for such antigenic diversity. Only one of them calls for mention at this stage.

If human beings had no tissue individuality, manifested by their histocompatibility antigens, and behaved like members of a pure-line strain of mice, cancer would be infectious from old persons in whom it appeared spontaneously to the young. Anyone who has followed the literature of tissue culture knows how 'infectious' cancer cell cultures can be in the laboratory. During the 1950s, far too many specially cherished cell lines turned out to be contaminated or replaced by the HeLa cells which were standard for most experiments at that period. I have contended that the existence in all mammalian species of a wide enough range of histocompatibility differences to ensure rejection of a homograft from any other individual of the species may have evolved from the need to ensure that cancer cells would not proliferate if they lodged, for example, on a mildly traumatized region of another individual, particularly on an infant. Every worker in experimental cancer research knows that a spontaneously appearing mouse tumour can usually be transplanted to another mouse of the same pure line. Attempts to transplant it to an unrelated animal always fail. This is in principle no different from the rejection of a normal skin graft from another mouse. All cancer cells, at least at the time of their first appearance as a tumour, carry the full battery of histocompatibility antigens of the individual animal involved.

For many years there had been a general belief that under favourable circumstances the body could develop some resistance to cancer and that this might be basically immunological in character. At the practical angle cancer immunity is only of interest when it can be manifested by the human or animal in which the tumour develops. This meant that anyone interested in the laboratory investigation of immune reactions in cancer had to carry out his search for tumour antigens, and antibodies or cell-mediated immunity, within a single pure-line stock of mice. Such work began in 1953 with Foley's demonstration[(149)] that tumours produced in pure-line mice with the carcinogen, methylcholanthrene (MCA), were antigenic. Experimental work with this system has now been active for twenty years, and with the development of pure strains of rats and guinea-pigs the basic findings have also been confirmed in these. By 1960 the general principles of cancer immunity in experimental animals had been established and increasing numbers of clinical investigators were applying related approaches to many types of human cancer.

In any age-associated random process there is no cut-off below some definite age. The age-specific incidence curve may be steep, but it extends down to an age far below that of the mean incidence. A significant fraction of the common cancers occur in young people at an age before their reproductive commitments have been completed. If that proportion became too large in any species, an evolutionary danger would exist and have to be overcome. The theme of this chapter is that such a danger does exist and has been overcome by the development of the process of immune (or immunological) surveillance.

Tumour-specific antigens

Before enquiring into the nature and clinical significance of immune surveillance, it is necessary to elaborate a little on the types of tumour-specific antigens and the immune responses they can provoke. In general, the demonstration that a mutant body cell, malignant or otherwise, can provoke an immune response leading to its destruction is interpreted as indicating that on the mutant cell surface new chemical configurations have appeared which are sufficiently different from any normal ones to be recognized as alien and provoke an immune response. Modern work on the nature of immunological tolerance and the complications introduced by the interactions of antigen with B-cells, T-cells, and antibody make their statement sound rather superficial, but it is fundamentally correct.

The nature of the new antigens has not been established in molecular terms, but at a biological level a good deal is known about them[150]. In the first place it is necessary to be clear that new tumour-specific transplantation antigens (TSTAs) have nothing in common with the histocompatibility antigens characteristic of all cells of the body, and initially at least of all cancer cells arising in it. The existence of individual differences in histocompatibility antigens means that in human patients significant immune reactions to a tumour can only be looked for in the blood and cells of the patient himself, though occasionally one meets a report in which an identical twin has provided useful information about the patient's immune reactions against his cancer.

Cancer immunity has in the last two decades become a very popular field for investigation, and like every other biological phenomenon it has developed new complexities with each increase in the number of investigators and the precision of their methods. At one stage one could think of *a* tumour-specific antigen. Now one is aware of many different ways by which cancer-specific antigens can be demonstrated *in vitro* as well as by the rather crude procedures by which tumour-specific transplantation antigens can be defined. All the modern techniques, from immunofluorescence to electronmicroscopy, have been applied. Two other sources of complexity and sometimes confusion must be mentioned. The first is the chemical dissection of the cell surface antigens in normal cells. Work is farthest advanced on the mouse lymphocyte, but if they were equally accessible to investigation other types of cell would doubtless provide an equal diversity of components. Then there are the complications which have appeared with the entry of tumour virologists into the field. The presence, whatever its significance, of virus, viral antigens, or fragments of the viral genome in cancer cells has added a new dimension of complexity to cancer immunity. No attempt to go into such detail would be appropriate here, but the implied reservations must be kept in mind in any simplified account of the three accepted types of tumour-specific antigen.

1. When a carcinogenic hydrocarbon, often MCA, is injected intra-

muscularly in pure-line mice or guinea-pigs, fibrosarcomatous tumours are produced with some regularity although the latent period can vary widely. Indirect evidence suggests that most or all of the tumours arise from a single cell. Antigenically they are strikingly diverse, both in their immunogenicity, i.e. their capacity to immunize against themselves, and in their specific antigen patterns. When a batch of antigenic tumours is obtained from up to sixteen genetically similar mice, each injected with the same preparation of MCA, all reports state that immunity is specific[151]. The tumour from mouse 1 can be used to immunize another dozen mice of the same strain and at the appropriate time all are challenged with active cells from tumours from mice 1, 2, 3 and 4. Only the cells from 1 will be rejected; 2, 3 and 4 will produce tumours. In all such experiments immunity is detected only against the cancer cell line used for immunization. Essentially similar findings are obtained in rats and guinea-pigs.

The origin of the new antigens is not known, and, as in all such phenomena, there are three main possibilities: (i) the antigens may result from changes induced directly by the carcinogen on the DNA, so modifying the structure of a cell surface component, (ii) the process of repair and normalization after a chemical lesion may have resulted in an error to be expressed phenotypically as an antigenic change, or (iii) the cell selected for malignant proliferation already carries the foreign antigen which has arisen by a mutational process before the injection was made.

Unless there are some new experimental approaches, it is probably impossible to choose between the alternatives. The sharpness of the specificity between tumour lines makes it almost certain that most or all of these MCA-induced tumours are monoclonal. This in turn suggests that only very rare cells can respond to the presence of the carcinogen and that these are premalignant cells under intrinsic mutagenic stimulation. Very rare individual cells carrying a new surface antigen will not provoke an immune response, but if a nodular clone containing millions of identical cells, each carrying the antigen, develops, an active series of cell-mediated and perhaps humoral immune responses can be expected. My reason for temporarily discarding this point of view was largely the report already mentioned[137] that single aneuploid prostate cells from C3H mice can be transformed by MCA and that fourteen clones, so produced, all showed unique antigenic qualities. The evidence would be much less cogent if each of the clones was derived from a cell in aneuploid premalignant form.

In any extensive experiment of this type the tumours obtained show a wide range of capacity to provoke an immune response and some show no demonstrable antigenicity at all. Such findings indicate that the development of a new antigen and of malignant qualities are not necessarily related. It is difficult to believe that some random impact of the carcinogenic agent on the DNA of a cell nucleus could *simultaneously* produce in an initially normal fibroblast two unrelated types of mutation without killing the cell. The only alternative is that the combination should arise as part of a pattern of intrinsic mutagenesis.

2. The second type of antigenic change is seen in experimental tumours induced by the standard oncogenic viruses, polyoma and SV40. When infection with either virus is induced in new-born mice or hamsters and tumours appear, these have a characteristic antigenicity which is currently interpreted as resulting from intrusion of viral DNA into the cell nucleus. Here it establishes an episomal relationship with the genome of the cell, so allowing the synthesis, by the cell, of some antigenic determinants characteristic of the virus. As would be expected, the changed antigenic character of a transformed and malignant cell clone is dominated by antigens coded by the viral genome, and except for minor antigenic difference, which must be specially sought, all tumours induced by polyoma have the same antigenicity but differ from that of SV40 tumours, which are again uniform among themselves.

The significance of viruses in relation to tumours is still the most active area of cancer research and one of the principal uses of the new U.S. funds for research on cancer will be in this field. There are viruses which produce proliferative lesions when transferred by natural means: human warts, rabbit papilloma and fibroma, Marek's disease of fowls. None of these conform at all closely to the pattern of human cancer. Under natural circumstances and in their natural hosts the conditions are not malignant, although Marek's disease can take on a much more actively lymphomatous form in one of the more susceptible breeds of fowls.

For obvious reasons most cancer research is done with viruses like polyoma and SV40, which have been adapted to produce tumours regularly in mice or hamsters on inoculation of a standard dose of virus. I have written extensively[152] on the artificial character of such research and stressed the immense selective power of laboratory transfer to produce any self-replicating variant of virus or cell that the experimenter is seeking consciously or unconsciously. For equally obvious reasons this attitude has not been popular and has had little influence on main line thought about cancer.

Malignant disease, even if we do not go beyond human clinical experience, is too complex a matter to allow any dogmatic statement. Undoubtedly environmental agents can greatly increase the incidence of certain types of cancer and there is no reason to exclude the possibility that some types of virus infection may also facilitate the emergence of some types of cancer. The most interesting situation is that involving the EB virus in man, which will be considered in some detail in Chapter 15, particularly in relation to Burkitt's lymphoma. Apart from this African tumour, the epidemiology of cancer gives no hint of an incidence pattern that could be easily related to microorganismal infection. If a virus is responsible for any of the common forms of human cancer, it must occupy a very different ecological niche from any of the classic pathogenic viruses. Until the viral oncologists have a much stronger case, I do not feel that anything is to be gained by discussing the behaviour of the laboratory cancer viruses. As far as human cancer study is concerned, they can for the time being be regarded as a shoal of red herrings.

3. Embryonic, foetal and ectopic antigens. Every somatic cell contains the whole genetic information of the zygote, most of it wholly unexpressed. It carries the coded instructions for synthesizing all primary constituents of the body, including those produced at any stage of life from conception to maturity. When malignancy is fully established, opportunites seem to arise with high frequency for the derepression of genes that were inactive in the normal cell line. The protein synthesized as a result may sometimes be recognized by its effect on the body generally if it is a potent hormone, but in most cases immunological approaches are necessary. When the abnormal 'ectopic' antigen is a substance commonly present in the blood, the only possible way of showing its production by the tumour is to isolate it from pure tumour cell cultures. If the antigen being liberated is characteristic of some normal organ but is there maintained in a form or situation that renders it inaccessible immunologically, it may provoke an autoimmune process directed against that organ and clinically diagnosable. Finally, we have the important situation, which may be characteristic of all tumours, that proteins characteristic of earlier (embryonic or foetal) stages of the somatic cell line may be produced. The frequency with which foetal antigens are found (and not always in malignant conditions) makes it likely that a process other than mutational is concerned. As the antigen has, by definition, been long absent from the body, it is operationally a foreign antigen and can provoke immune responses. There is as yet little evidence that foetal antigens in a tumour can function as TSTAs. The

two best known examples, the α-foeto-protein of liver tumours and the carcino-embryonic antigen of colonic carcinomas, have little or no antigenicity in the patients concerned and are detected as antigen circulating in the blood as well as being present in the cells of the tumour. Several authors have failed to find evidence that a foetal antigen known to be present in an experimental tumour could serve as a TSTA and induce its rejection(153).

The evidence for a surveillance function

The idea of immune surveillance was suggested in 1957 in terms of the possibility 'that small accumulations of tumour cells may develop and because of their possession of new antigenic potentialities provoke an effective immunological reaction with regression of the tumour and no clinical hint of its existence'(109). This can still be taken as a definition of the process. The concept is one which can probably never be unequivocally demonstrated in man, and many people have doubted its existence. The striking crop of malignancies that have been reported in patients, mostly well below the cancer age, under immunosuppressive therapy after kidney transplantation has recently swung opinion in its favour. So, too, has the occurrence of tumours, and especially lymphoreticular sarcomas in children suffering from immunodeficiency diseases of relatively chronic character, such as the Wiskott–Aldrich syndrome and ataxia-telangiectasia.

At the experimental level I find the most illuminating experience in Prehn's analysis of the results of injecting a large series of mice with a standard dose of MCA(154). Of eighty-eight tumours that were analysed, eight were scored as of high antigenicity, thirty of low immunogenicity, and fifty as non-immunizing. The incubation period varied with the antigenicity. All the highly antigenic tumours appeared within fifteen days, and the nine tumours which appeared after thirty days were all non-immunogenic. The implication is strong that, unless an incipient tumour with high immunogenicity can overcome the immune response by its active growth, it will fail to develop, while non-antigenic tumours can grow slowly and become evident at a much later stage. The other conclusion to be drawn is that the existence and immunogenicity of the tumour-specific antigen has no bearing on the malignancy of the tumour; it is an epiphenomenon.

Prehn's results may also have a significant bearing on the origin of the diversity of the tumour-specific antigens found in these experiments.

The possibility has already been favoured that these antigens may be pre-existent in the cell that initiated the tumour. It is inevitable that many silent somatic mutations must occur for every one that leads to a demonstrable end result. Mutations giving rise to antigenic change in components of the cell membrane of fibroblasts could be quite common, and, being at random, a very wide diversity of antigenic patterns is to be expected. As long as the number of cells with one specific pattern is small, they will attract no attention from the immune system. Effective antigenicity would depend on the development of a large enough clone to provide an adequate dose of the new antigen. A prima facie case for or against this hypothesis could be made from experiments similar to those of Prehn, in which mice of a wide range of ages were used. If the antigenic patterns arise by silent somatic mutation, the proportion of immunogenic tumours should rise with age.

Reverting to the more theoretical aspects of the relation between ageing and cancer, we can look first at the question of whether immune surveillance has any evolutionary significance or, like cancer itself, is a mere by-product of processes which have. It is wholly unrealistic to raise the question of how many tumours would arise, and when, in an otherwise normal individual who had no immune capacity against any tumour that might be initiated. Obviously this would mean a complete absence of the T-immune system, with death of the patient before any tumours could be recognized. In all conditions which, with or without maintenance treatment, can survive for ten or more years, the immune system may be functioning far below normal levels of effectiveness, but it has some capacity or the patient could not survive. In ataxia-telangiectasia and Wiskott–Aldrich syndrome the death rate from cancer is something over 10 per cent, mainly in people under twenty, with a high proportion due to malignant tumours of the lymphoid tissues. It is fair enough to say that immune surveillance is *one* of the important functions of the immune system, but the possibility of its being no more than an activity necessarily related to a primary evolutionary need in other directions is far from excluded.

The need to eliminate foreign cells not very grossly different from those of the body has already been mentioned and in different contexts I have discussed the three situations that are likely to have been important in its evolution. They are the need to prevent cancer cells being infectious to children, the need to control the potential invasiveness of the embryo in all forms of viviparous reproduction, and the dangers of parasitism by closely related species. All have the common requirement of a system by which the cells of any other individual intruding into the body's tissues can be recognized as different. Any solution adopted must necessarily be a two-sided system to provide both a diversity of patterns to be recognized and a mechanism for their recognition. 'Self', in other words chemical patterns genetically proper to the body, must be differentiated from 'not-self'. The existing mechanism, essentially the T-immune system, is obviously precisely what is needed to deal with any foreign cells and at the same time with any cells arising in the body which carry new antigens, always provided these are produced in sufficient amount to provoke an effective immune response.

Does immune surveillance significantly modify the age-specific incidence of cancer?

I can see no immediate way to assess quantitatively what part immune surveillance plays in determining the incidence of cancer. On general grounds one would assume that any effect would be very small prenatally but would rise rapidly after birth and perhaps reach a maximum about the age of twelve but with a long plateau extending into middle age before a steady fall became noticeable. Such a control would, however, have to work against a cancer-initiating process which on any type of reasonable scheme would build up progressively with age. This would be the case if environmental carcinogens acting over long periods were wholly responsible, and equally if cumulative somatic mutation was the sole agent. It would hold too for any sort of logical compromise between the two. The difficulties of interpreting the cigarette-lung cancer situation indicate how far we are from getting the process of carcinogenesis into quantitative form. Until that is done it will be impossible to make more than speculative estimates as to how far surveillance prevents the emergence of overt and fatal cancer.

In Figure 17 I have shown a log-log plot of all cancers other than leukaemias and lymphomas as recorded in England and Wales, and added two possible curves that might represent the age-specific incidence of these cancers in the absence of immune surveillance. The first and most extreme suggestion is based on the assumption that childhood cancers, including leukaemia, are initiated by the standard process of intrinsic mutagenesis and are conspicuous only because their critical initiatory stage coincides with the foetal period of minimal or zero immune reactivity. An extension of the early childhood peak in the

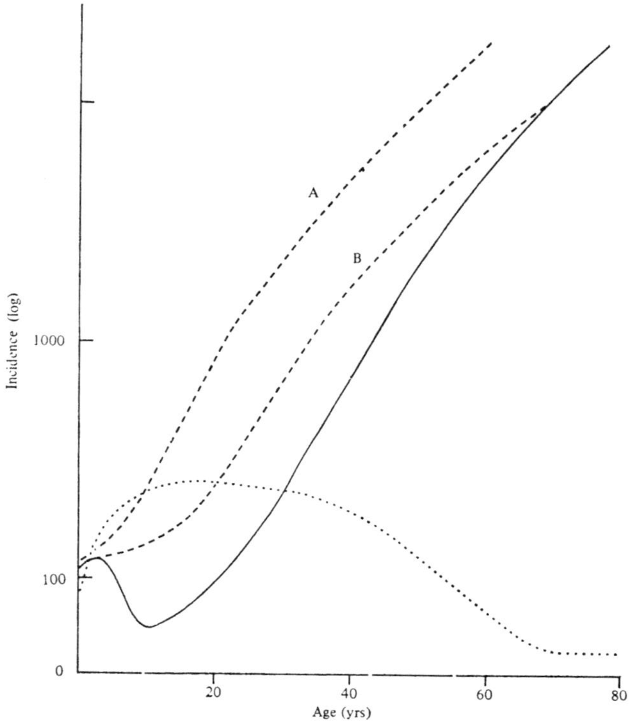

Figure 17 A speculative indication of the effect of surveillance. The heavy line shows the age-specific incidence of all tumours except leukaemias etc., the dotted line gives an indication of the probable effectiveness of the immune response at ages, while the broken lines A and B could indicate the incidence of cancer in the absence of effective immune surveillance (see text)

standard straight line at a slope of 5 would make cancer by far the main cause of death and the principal determinant of average lifespan.

In discussing the question of foetal radiation and the childhood cancers and leukaemias, I mentioned the opinion that there was some special susceptibility to the initiation of cancer in prenatal life even without any demonstrable impact from the environment. When one considers the well known evidence that many neuroblastomas regress simply as a result of the maturation of the still immature malignant neuroblasts, it becomes very difficult to regard any type of cancer-producing mechanism as persisting essentially the same from conception to maturity and old age.

The second curve is based on the assumption that all childhood cancers under five, and possibly all under ten, are initiated in foetal life, where in addition to a virtual absence of immune response we assume a strong 'promoting' factor which disappears soon after birth. On the assumption that immune surveillance is at an approximate plateau of efficiency from five to fifty and thereafter diminishes, the level of incidence might rise to give over the twenty to fifty age period about the incidence found for non-lymphoid tumours in patients under immunosuppression. Curve 2 can be regarded as a reasonable guess of what might be expected without immune surveillance, with the proviso made previously that complete elimination of the relevant immune functions would almost certainly be incompatible with life.

The part played by immune surveillance in leukaemia and lymphomatous conditions has not been considered here in view of the quite different age incidence curves and the indication of a 350-fold increase in the incidence of malignant lymphomas or reticulum cell sarcomas in immunosuppressed patients or individuals with some immunodeficiency diseases. The general theme will be looked at in the next chapter.

CHAPTER 15

LYMPHORETICULAR MALIGNANCIES AND THEIR RELATION TO HERPESVIRUS INFECTIONS

There has been very great recent interest in a field of study which superficially has only a remote relationship to the phenomena of ageing but which must be relevant to the overall concepts being developed. It concerns malignant tumours and leukaemias derived from cells of the lymphoid series and their frequent association with viruses of the herpesvirus group[155]. If changes in the lymphocyte–immunocyte cell lines are basic to ageing, any characteristic qualities of maliginancy in these lines must be to some degree relevant and call for explanation.

The lymphoreticular malignancies

There is a wide range of lymphomatous conditions to be considered, of which the best known are Hodgkin's disease, lymphosarcoma, Burkitt's lymphoma, acute leukaemia, chronic lymphatic leukaemia, multiple myeloma, and the various monoclonal gammopathies without solid tumour. It is usual both in experimental animals and human patients to include tumours diagnosed histologically as reticulum cell sarcomas with frankly lymphomatous tumours. This has found recent justification in work by Stein *et al.*[156] on the production of immunoglobulins by human tumour cell lines in culture. Cells from four tumours diagnosed histologically as reticulum cell sarcomas all produced IgM. Two of them had in fact been clinically associated with a Waldenström type monoclonal macroglobulinaemia in the patients from whom they were derived. It will probably soon be legitimate to regard all the lymphoreticular malignancies as immunoblastomas and to look forward to the time when T-cell tumours can be defined as clearly as those derived from the immunoglobulin producers of the B series.

Lymphoreticular malignancies (LRM) differ in their age incidence from most other cancers. Acute leukaemias of stem cell type are essentially conditions of childhood, while chronic lymphatic leukaemia has almost the same age incidence as a typical cancer, but there are cases with cells of intermediate types and a range of younger adult cases to fill in the gaps. Lymphosarcoma, lymphoma, and Hodgkin's disease may occur at any age, but include many children and young adults. The most interesting feature of these LRM from the present point of view is their great preponderance among the lethal or life-threatening tumours that appear in persons with immunodeficiency diseases or who are under prolonged treatment with immunosuppressive drugs.

In the presumably genetic immunodeficiency diseases a recent review[(157)] shows that seventy-seven of the ninety-three malignant neoplasms on record fell into this category. Lymphomatous tumours are also conspicuous among the lethal tumours arising in transplant patients under immunosuppressive drug treatment. The most recent compilation by Hoover and Fraumeni[(158)] records fourteen cases of reticulum cell sarcoma in reports of 6297 transplants. They calculate that this is about 350 times the reported incidence of tumours so diagnosed in a normal population of the same age distribution. In view of differences in criteria used for diagnosis, this ratio may be unduly high, but even comparing the whole group of LRM the incidence is thirty-five times that in the controls.

In both groups, of persons with immunodeficiency disease and transplant patients under immunosuppression, a variety of other tumours, including the common types of carcinoma, are observed at a higher incidence than normal though with a much smaller relative excess than of lymphomatous tumours.

There is a fairly wide consensus of opinion that the excess of tumours is due to a failure or weakness of the normal function of immunological surveillance. What has not been explained satisfactorily is the excess of malignancies of lymphoreticular origin. In seeking hypotheses, the first approach on general grounds would be to assume that lymphoid cell malignancies are frequently initiated, perhaps more frequently than in any other cell type, particularly at younger ages, and that, normally, immunological surveillance is very effective in eliminating malignant clones at an early stage.

To substantiate that hypothesis will require some discussion (*a*) of the evidence suggesting a high level of initiated malignancy in lymphocytes, and (*b*) of the justification for regarding immune surveillance as particularly effective against lymphocytes with aberrant antigens of any sort.

Liability to malignant change

Before considering any special role of viruses in the initiation of human neoplastic conditions involving lymphoid cells it is expedient first to compare their epidemiological features, particularly sex and age-specific incidence, with those of the common epithelial malignancies. The standard form of these curves has been discussed at length in Chapter 12, and the first point to be made is that two important conditions of the LRM group, multiple myelomatosis and chronic lymphatic leukaemia, conform almost precisely to that pattern. Cells of the lymphocyte series are clearly as subject to the standard process by which cancer is generated as any other clonally proliferating lines.

Other malignant and semi-malignant conditions show quite different curves. Acute leukaemia is mainly a childhood disease, Hodgkin's disease one of middle life (Figure 18). If these conditions are generated by intrinsic mutagenesis, some special lability not seen in other cell lines must be playing a part. Much has still to be learnt about the potentialities of the human lymphocyte, but there is already ample evidence of its immense genetic lability as a somatic cell. No matter how large a complement of genes controlling immunoglobulin structure is present in the zygote, a highly complex programme of activation, intragenic recombination, accelerated point mutation and phenotypic restriction, or some equivalent series of processes, must be completed before a specific T or B clone can come into being. Every new development in cellular immunology in the last decade seems to have made a fresh demand for genetically based adjustment to subserve new functions. I have recently suggested, for example[159], that the transfer factor of Lawrence associated with T-cell function must call for a programme of diversification and phenotypic restriction analogous to the differentiation of specific antibody-producing clones. To these physiological changes can be added the great variety of autoimmune cell clones, both T and B, of very diverse aggressiveness, and the hyperactive but not otherwise malignant clones of antibody-producing cells giving rise to the monoclonal gammopathies of Waldenström.

This is surely enough to indicate an exceptional genetic lability, and

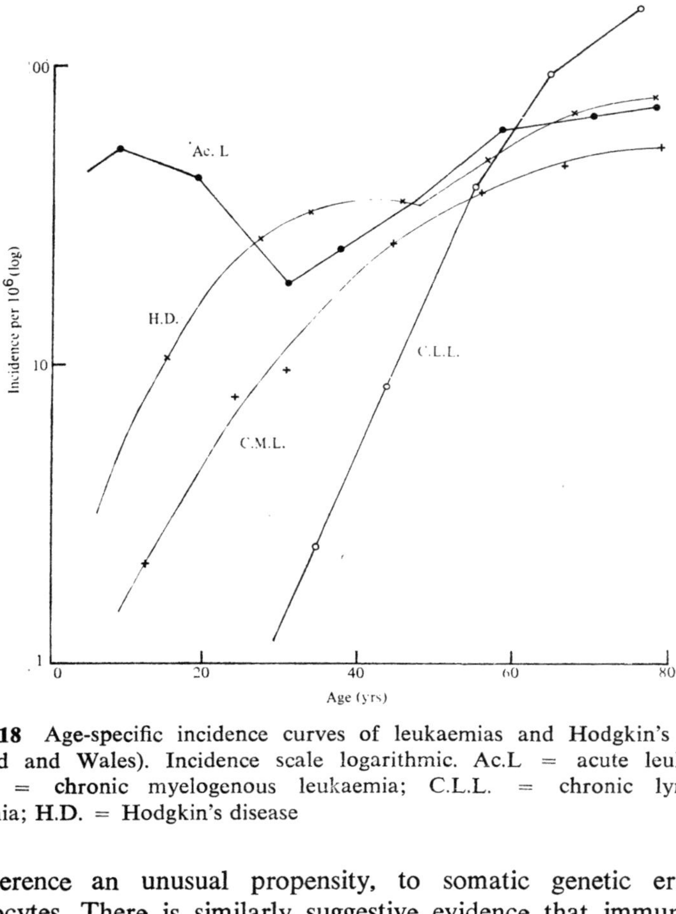

Figure 18 Age-specific incidence curves of leukaemias and Hodgkin's disease (England and Wales). Incidence scale logarithmic. Ac.L = acute leukaemia; C.M.L. = chronic myelogenous leukaemia; C.L.L. = chronic lymphatic leukaemia; H.D. = Hodgkin's disease

by inference an unusual propensity, to somatic genetic error in lymphocytes. There is similarly suggestive evidence that immune surveillance may be specially effective against lymphocytes carrying recognizably foreign antigenic determinants.

Special susceptibility to immune surveillance

Jerne[160] has recently presented an attractive picture of the immune system as a multidimensional eigen-system of interlocking interaction and mutual control amongst cells and antibodies. One point specially emphasized by Jerne is that each antibody or immune cell receptor has of necessity a foreign configuration, an *idiotope*, in the specific structure of the V segments of immunoglobulin that confer the individuality on the macromolecules. For the purely physiological functions of the immune system it is essential that an enormous population of lymphocytes with their surface T- or B-receptors and antigens should have adequate facilities to make transient contact with the largest possible number of other lymphocytes and with any cell types liable to be carrying foreign antigens on their surface, notably the dendritic macrophages of lymphoid tissue. Everything that is known about the questing motility of lymphocytes, the very rapid movement in and out of lymph nodes and other accumulations of lymphoid tissue, and the distribution of dendritic phagocytic cells, indicates that this requirement is more than adequately fulfilled. If a lymphocyte carries a mutant pattern on a cell membrane protein it will have every chance of meeting one or more of the lymphocytes which in virtue of their immune receptors can recognize the foreign pattern and react to it by proliferation or some other appropriate reaction. To recognize a similarly alien pattern on an epithelial or other fixed cell type will call a much more indirect and inefficient set of processes into action.

It will be equally evident that any lymphocytes cytotoxic for a recognizable mutant form will have a greater opportunity of making effective contact with the target cell if it is a lymphocyte than with any other type. A capacity to eliminate any unwanted type of lymphocyte may in fact be regarded as one of the body's prime needs for survival, and a special efficiency of immune surveillance against incipient lymphocytic malignancy is only to be expected.

The herpesviruses associated with LRM

An approach of this sort to lymphoreticular malignancy, in which concepts of somatic mutation and immunological interactions are alone operative, will impress most workers in the field as very old-fashioned. I am well aware that contemporary discussion of the various lymphomatous conditions found in man, monkeys, mice and chickens is dominated by consideration of the viruses frequently associated with them. It is conventional to ascribe all the neoplastic aspects to the results of virus infection. A good case, in fact an apparently irrefutable case, for this point of view is presented by Klein in recent reviews[151, 161–163]. There is, however, one major discrepancy in the argument. The African tumour (Burkitt's lymphoma) has been shown to be almost regularly monoclonal in character, derived from a single changed cell[164]. This is not the behaviour of a viral disease but of a condition arising by somatic mutation. The fact in itself may justify re-exploration of the discarded hypothesis that viral infection can only induce overt malignancy by making use of somatic mutational changes that precede infection. Before developing this point of view it is necessary to outline the relationship of herpesviruses to lymphoreticular malignancies and related conditions. Klein has had special interest in the bearing of this field on immune surveillance, and I shall make much use of his material.

The mammalian viruses which can provoke or are regularly associated with LRM are predominantly herpesviruses. They include Epstein–Barr virus (EBV), which is almost certainly the etiological agent in infectious mononucleosis as well as being found regularly in all human lymphoid cell lines that are capable of growing indefinitely in cell culture. All cases of Burkitt's lymphoma show evidence of infection with EBV (as do a majority of Africans in the same regions) and the virus has been experimentally detected in many of the tumours. Nasopharyngeal carcinoma, a predominantly Asian condition, is the only other neoplasm in which it is found with some frequency.

Herpesvirus saimiri is now known to be a harmless inhabitant of the South American squirrel monkey. Squirrel monkeys shed the virus and develop antibody, but no tumours. Marmosets and owl monkeys, also New World forms, are never found harbouring the virus, and when it is injected they regularly develop lethal lymphomas. All three species develop antibody after primary infection, but the squirrel monkey at ten to twelve days, as compared with twenty to fifty days in the other two species.

Marek's disease of the chicken, also due to a herpesvirus, is readily spread and infects a high proportion of birds. The frequency of malignant lymphomatous tumours, however, varies much between chicken strains. In resistant strains benign infections are the rule, but the incidence of tumours can be greatly increased in such strains by neonatal thymectomy. A high degree of immunity can be induced in susceptible strains by immunization with a non-pathogenic turkey strain of the virus.

The role of EBV

Human infections with EBV have been much more deeply studied than any of the others and are clearly the only ones that are relevant enough to the general theme to need discussion. The conventional virological interpretation can be found in any recent text book and in Klein's reviews. The alternative approach could take the following form.

From the point of view of clinical science, the main significance of EBV is as the etiological agent of the commonest form of infectious mononucleosis. Specific antibody tests indicate that infection by the virus is extremely common in all the human populations that have been examined. We can safely assume that EBV is a highly successful virus, well adapted to its human host species. Everything suggests that the standard interaction of virus and host takes the form of infection in infancy or early childhood. Such infections are not associated with mononucleosis and are presumably symptomless or mildly febrile episodes with some multiplication of the virus and re-liberation in saliva to continue the chain of infection. Two persisting changes follow infection. Antibody against viral antigens develops and persists indefinitely; its presence is an unequivocal index of insusceptibility to infectious mononucleosis. The second indicator of past infection is based on the regular finding that all human lymphocyte cultures that can be carried on indefinitely are carriers of EBV in the sense that a proportion of the cells show evidence of viral components. It appears that a certain proportion of lymphocytes become carriers during the primary infantile infection, and by some unknown mechanism sufficient new cells become infected to maintain some carrier cells indefinitely.

Mononucleosis is predominantly a disease of adolescents and young adults who have not been infected in infancy and have initially no antibody. Here the requirement is to interpret the leukaemia-like proliferation of lymphocytes, the rather extraordinary range of immunological manifestations, and the almost invariable complete recovery. Perhaps of almost equal importance is the existence of clinically almost indistinguishable syndromes associated with cytomegalovirus infection and systemic toxoplasmosis in adults.

Following the indication from the predominance of lymphoma-type malignancies in conditions of immunodeficiency, we assume that lymphocytes are subject to a relatively high level of somatic mutation and are more vulnerable to surveillance type control than any other class of cells. At any period of life there will be a proportion of mutants in circulation, and according to the standard rules cells with more than one mutation will increase with age. When infection with EBV occurs, we accept that its initial form is, as in infants, non-cytopathogenic infection of lymphocytes with an occasional cell breaking down and liberating virus. Leukaemoid proliferation leading to the diagnosis of infectious mononucleosis is ascribed to infection of a premalignant cell which has probably accumulated two or more sequential mutations, the infection providing a trigger to release the latent proliferative change. The hypothesis has the testable implication that the abnormal cells in a typical infectious mononucleosis case should occasionally be monoclonal and always no more than oligoclonal. The younger the subject, the more likely one would be to demonstrate a monoclonal lymphocytosis.

No one has provided an adequate interpretation of the wide range of heterophile antibodies and autoantibodies that may be found in association with the leukaemoid population of lymphocytes. This is a fascinating problem, especially when it is remembered that current opinion regards the atypical lymphocytes as T-cells. The finding may well be related to the fact that most 'tolerance' is more a function of T-cells than B-cells, but it would hardly be relevant to expand that suggestion in the present context. What is more apropos is that the modified lymphocytes characteristic of infectious mononucleosis are readily grown in cell culture and, like other lymphoid cell lines carrying EBV, are abnormally reactive in mixed lymphocyte reactions, even with normal lymphocytes from the same individual donor when it is practical to make the experiment. In line with the genetic lability of lymphocytes one can assume that the abnormal forms have sufficient antigenic differences from the normal population to provoke immune responses, probably both humoral and cellular. This becomes eventually a highly effective immune surveillance operation, so effective in fact that only on the rarest occasions does an infectious mononucleosis end as an acute leukaemia. In the great majority who recover, persisting infection with EBV in a few non-responsive cells is the only sequel, leaving the position essentially the same as follows infantile infection.

The experimental evidence is clear that Burkitt's lymphoma occurs only in children who have been infected with EBV and that all cell culture lines derived from the tumours can be shown to carry virus or virus-related antigens. EBV infection is almost equally common in all the human populations studied, so that some explanation is needed for the limitation of typical Burkitt's lymphoma to Africa and New Guinea. Burkitt believes that the difference is related to the universal (holoepidemic) presence of malaria in the regions involved(165). In the malarial child with a very large spleen there is obvious lymphocytic proliferation giving a population in which more somatic mutants than usual can accumulate, including some which by hypothesis can be triggered to proliferate by EBV. Add to this the known immunodepression associated with malaria and the likelihood that in young children there are preferred regions where a stimulated lymphocyte in the presence of an incompletely effective immune response can proliferate to a solid monoclonal lymphoma.

Hodgkin's disease

At the risk of intruding into a very well studied field, one can hardly avoid looking at the etiology of Hodgkin's disease in the light of this work on EBV infections and associated lymphomatous conditions.

The epidemiology of Hodgkin's disease has some quite striking geographical variations, shown particularly in the age distribution of cases. An extensive survey of many parts of the world has recently been published and the results summarized by Corea and O'Conor[166]. In Central America and tropical Africa it is reported to be predominantly a disease of children, with very few examples among young adults or older people. In the United States and Western Europe there is no significant incidence in young children, but a well marked young adult incidence, with a peak at 25–30 and a low point at 45–50, after which there is a steady rise

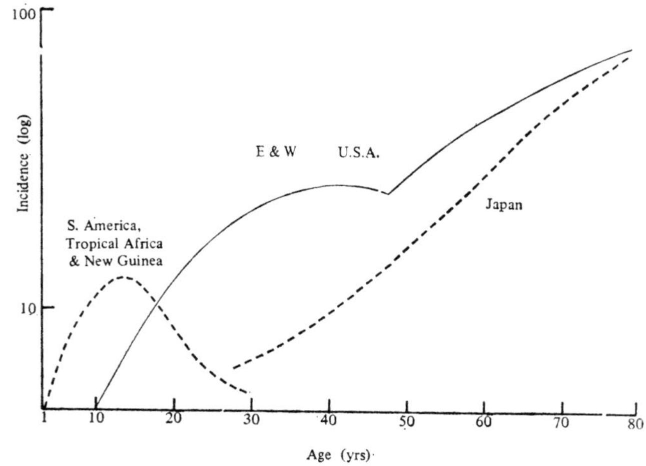

Figure 19 Schematic illustration of the age-specific incidence of Hodgkin's disease in contrasting environments. In primitive tropical regions most cases are under twenty, in affluent developed communities there is a well marked young adult incidence as well as a major age-associated group. In Japan neither the childhood nor the young adult component is seen

to old age of typical malignant type. In Japan neither childhood nor young adult incidence is seen, the incidence being that of a typical age-associated malignancy. As Cole[167] and others have emphasized, this epidemiological pattern is unlike any other malignancy, but has obvious analogies to the behaviour of several infectious conditions. There has therefore been considerable interest in the possibility that Hodgkin's disease, at least in the young adult form, could be a result of EBV infection. The possibility seems to have been adequately studied and excluded by Goldman and Aisenberg[168]. Comparing sera from fifty-seven patients with Hodgkin's disease and a comparable control series, they found essentially identical distributions of antibodies against EBV, herpes simplex 1 and cytomegalovirus. The evidence therefore eliminates any possibility that EBV has an analogous role in Hodgkin's to that in infectious mononucleosis and Burkitt's lymphoma.

Two important findings, however, must be kept in mind. In a proportion of cases of infectious mononucleosis[169] and Burkitt lymphoma[170] cells histologically identical with the Reed–Sternberg cells of Hodgkin's disease are present. That particular cell morphology is not therefore specific for Hodgkin's disease; it may well point to some common feature in the pathogenesis of the three conditions. Then we must remember that EBV is not the only infectious agent that can provoke the clinical picture of infectious mononucleosis in man. Cytomegalovirus[171, 171a] and primary toxoplasmosis[172] can do so, and there could be others. If the epidemiological pattern of Hodgkin's disease calls for a process analogous to what has been postulated for infectious mononucleosis or Burkitt's lymphoma, it would be quite in order to consider the possible activity of a widespread virus generally resembling EBV but serologically distinct. The point can be given more force by remembering that in the absence of Burkitt's lymphoma there is no likelihood whatever that the etiology of infectious mononucleosis would have been elucidated.

As one with a good deal of past experience in viral epidemiology, I believe that the age characteristic of Hodgkin's disease in different parts of the world must indicate that one component of its etiology can only be a widespread low grade infectious agent, presumably a virus. I shall therefore assume that there exists a Hodgkin's disease virus (HDV), specific for man, not cytopathic in standard cell cultures, transmitted by contact or droplet infection, and in the great majority of infections producing no symptoms. In addition one must postulate as well the special quality that the virus can stimulate lymphocytes already on the way towards malignancy to take on active malignant or quasi-malignant proliferation, and for one or more such cells to find an anatomical niche where they can resist any surveillance-type immune response against them. An hypothesis of that sort can be seen to imply the following consequences in the three types of human environment that are distinguished by Corea and O'Conor.

1. Primitive cultural conditions in Africa and South America— Here the dominant factor is likely to be the intense prevalence of infection in early childhood. Malaria and other relatively massive infections will make heavy demands on lymphocytic turnover and allow the unduly early appearance of premalignant mutants within the lymphocyte population. At the same time one is almost bound to postulate nearly universal early infection and immunization with HDV. There will be virtually complete immunization against any later initiation of Hodgkin's disease, but, as with EBV and Burkitt's lymphoma, there will be a very small proportion of children who develop the disease a few years later. There will be little or no later cases of Hodgkin's disease.

2. Japan—where population is dense and infection must spread easily but children are well nourished and there are good public health services. There is essentially no juvenile or young adult Hodgkin's disease. The simplest interpretation is that infection with HDV is nearly universal in childhood, but in well nourished, basically healthy children it has no more than an immunizing effect. When a lymphomatous condition, age-associated Hodgkin's disease, develops, any residual infection with HDV is of little significance compared to the effect of cumulative mutation and the diminishing efficiency of immune surveillance, both age-associated conditions.

3. United States—here there is a well marked young adult peak of Hodgkin's disease, which for the most part is relatively amenable to treatment, as well as the more malignant age-associated variety. It is also of interest that 'young' Hodgkin's disease is markedly less common in the south-eastern states than in the north-eastern—just as adolescent poliomyelitis was in the 1930s and 1940s.

As with infectious mononucleosis, one assumes that in affluent areas a substantial proportion of young children miss infection and immunization with HDV. Those non-immune are subject to infection in young adult life, probably under the same circumstances as EBV. Either the necessary accumulation of mutations is much rarer or the likelihood of effective infection lower than for infectious mononucleosis. As in infectious mononucleosis, most of the infected cells are eventually eliminated immunologically, but in the subjects in whom Hodgkin's disease will develop, an occasional cell finds a privileged microenvironment within lymphoid tissue. There have been suggestions that the thymus is a common initial site of Hodgkin's disease, but all that is required is that the stimulated cell should settle down in a region where it is relatively or absolutely insusceptible to an active immune response. It is possible that this only occurs in that small proportion of people who have a minor genetically based inefficiency of the T-immune system.

The age-associated Hodgkin's disease also characteristic of the United States can be most readily interpreted as a malignant condition in which HDV plays a minimal or no part. One would expect to find that most had been infected with HDV, and, by analogy with EBV, persisting evidence of viral antigens might be found. It seems adequate, however, to ascribe activation of the malignant process to some other trigger and to believe that the immune response is directed more against the mutant antigens than HDV antigens. As judged by the therapeutic result, the immune response is very ineffective and the disease pursues a typical malignant course.

Immunological features of Hodgkin's disease

For many years clinicians and pathologists have recognized that Hodgkin's disease was very different from any standard malignant disease. When tuberculosis was commoner than now, the almost constant association of Hodgkin's disease with tuberculosis was often commented on. It was also recognized that most patients gave a negative tuberculin test. Modern elaboration of these findings has led to the recognition that there is a gross deficiency of cell-mediated (T-system) immunity in the disease. Patients tested with a battery of five or six microorganismal antigens (tuberculin, diphtheria toxoid, etc.), to which most normal adults would give three or four positive reactions, will show none or one or two weak reactions[(173)]. More direct tests of capacity to develop sensitization also show gross deficiency in patients with active disease. Aisenberg[(174)] used the chemical dinitrochlorobenzene to induce skin sensitization. Of twenty-five active cases of Hodgkin's disease, none were sensitized, compared with 100 per cent of normal controls and eleven out of twelve patients with inactive or recovered Hodgkin's disease. Test of ability to reject donor skin grafts showed more than 50 per cent of Hodgkin's disease patients retaining the graft for more than thirty days.

As indicated earlier, a patient with active Hodgkin's disease, known to have given a positive tuberculin test before the onset of his disease and now non-reactive, may recover skin reactivity when the disease is checked. There is often some months' delay from the time of clinical improvement after therapy to the return of skin sensitivity. Passive transfer of leucocytes from a tuberculin-positive but otherwise normal individual also fails to produce local or general sensitization to tuberculin in a patient with active Hodgkin's disease. It is obviously necessary to assume that most of the immune deficiency is a result of the disease rather than one of the factors in its induction. The condition in some ways resembles the disappearance of a positive tuberculin reaction for a few weeks after an attack of measles, and any explanation must be looked for in immunological terms. It is highly relevant that irregular, often severe fever is usually seen in Hodgkin's disease and that amyloid degeneration is common in later stages.

In discussing measles some years ago[(175)], I ascribed the inhibition of T-cell immunity to the immune interaction of two sets of lymphocytes, cells carrying virus and/or viral antigens on their surface, and immunocytes reactive against viral antigens. At the height of the measles rash and fever there is widespread liberation of lymphokines and mutual destruction of lymphocytes, involving apparently a wide range of cells not specifically implicated in the interaction. It makes sense to look at developed Hodgkin's disease as a subacute manifestation of essentially the same process. By hypothesis the proliferating cells are (*a*) malignant in virtue of preceding somatic mutation and (*b*) subject to stimulating non-cytopathic infection with HDV. Both changes can be assumed to provide new antigens to be carried on the cell surface of the proliferating cells and these will provoke a predominantly T-cell response. The difference from measles or infectious mononucleosis (EBV) is that in these the elimination of the cells carrying foreign antigens is effectively complete, while in Hodgkin's disease a proportion of the pathogenic cells remain inaccessible or invulnerable to the immune attack. A persisting fluctuating equilibrium between 'attack' and 'defence' would give a rationale for the whole clinical and pathological picture of young adult Hodgkin's disease.

The effectiveness of immune surveillance

As Klein emphasizes, the whole natural history of infectious mononucleosis and Burkitt lymphoma points to the striking effectiveness of immune surveillance against abnormal lymphocytes. One might also add that it points as well to the very frequent appearance of antigenic variants on lymphocyte surfaces that call for surveillance action.

This brings us rather directly back to the phenomenon with which this chapter opened: the predominance of lymphoreticular malignancies in patients with immunodeficiency disease or under immunosuppressive drug therapy. Everything points to the initial hypothesis being correct, that in younger people potentially malignant lymphocyte mutants are common, but even when triggered into activity by tolerated infection are readily eliminated by a highly effective surveillance function. It is when that function is below an effective level for either genetic or pharmacological reasons that surveillance breaks down and tumours become increasingly frequent.

If the approach I have used is correct, it has an number of interesting offshoots that might be explored, but the only ones relevant to the general theme of ageing are in relation to autoimmune disease.

1. The first concerns the high frequency with which monoclonal antibody proteins react with autoantigens or with haptens which are likely to be sterically related to accessible antigenic determinants of body components. An autoimmune clone is by hypothesis one which has undergone more than one somatic mutation on its line of descent, and it is also one which is chronically stimulated to proliferation. It is therefore a favoured candidate for an additional mutation which will push it to neoplastic activity and give rise to myelomatosis or Waldenström's macroglobulinaemia.

2. The probability that autoimmune clones are subject to immune surveillance is considerably increased and it may become necessary to find additional reasons why some autoimmune clones persist, particularly in young people. The most likely one is that either the aberrant immunocyte line has no 'new' antigenic determinants or—which is almost the same thing—that the repertoire of immunocytes available includes none with complementarily patterned receptors capable of significant binding to the presumed new antigens on the pathogenic cells. A related matter which could justify research is to determine whether abnormal receptors or antibody characteristic of an autoimmune clone manifest idiotypic specificity based on the *antigenic* quality of the VL or VH segments (antibody-specific) of the immunoglobulin.

All things considered, it seems legitimate to accept the conclusion that one of the mechanisms available to prevent or damp down the activity of pathogenic autoimmune clones of immunocytes is immune surveillance.

Some related aspects of cancer

The role of environmental factors in cancer was discussed in Chapter 13 in regard to some of the commoner sites of epithelial tumours. Something more may be said about two of these sites, the skin and the cervix uteri, in the light of the EBV role in lymphomatous tumours.

Skin epithelium is a tissue which persists in its continuing clonal proliferation through life. As in any such tissue, somatic mutations of neutral or negative survival value will accumulate with age; lethal mutations or sequences of mutation that lead to error catastrophe will gradually reduce the number of basal epidermal cells. Exposure to ultraviolet light, sunburn, leads to excessive production of new epidermis, and we can reasonably assume the same progressive dwindling of a 'quota of cell generations'. A man of my age has only to look at the backs of his hands to see the thinning of the epidermis with here and there localized hyperkeratoses of piled up epidermal epithelium to recognize the logical consequences of that interpretation.

It is evident enough that sequential mutations with an overall proliferative advantage are responsible for the hyperkeratoses which are so commonly seen in Australia, and almost equally so for the rarer basal cell carcinomas (rodent ulcers) which are the commonest type of skin malignancy. The point to be emphasized is that there is no necessary direct carcinogenic effect of ultraviolet light involved. Thymic dimerizations, and possibly other types of chemical damage to DNA, will be numerous and in the course of their repair there are bound to be errors. The resulting mutational effects, random in quality as always, will include some leading towards malignancy.

In Australia, which has more sunshine than any other region predominantly occupied by people of north European ancestry, there is special interest in skin cancer, particularly basal cell carcinoma and malignant melanoma. Kidney transplantation is well developed at all the major surgical centres, and extensive experience of tumours arising in patients under prolonged immunosuppression has been accumulated. The most significant finding has been the large number of instances in which carcinoma of the skin has developed from pre-existing hyperkeratoses, particularly on the backs of the hands[176, 177]. The tumours are squamous-celled epitheliomas which, compared to basal cell tumours, are relatively uncommon in Australia.

The interpretation of this result in terms of immunosurveillance is considerably less straightforward than the situation with lymphomatous conditions. One is almost bound to postulate that under normal conditions any invasive proliferation by a hyperkeratotic clone of epidermic cells is effectively attacked, presumably by T-cells, as soon as it intrudes into vascularized tissue. The behaviour of kerato-acanthomas, which quite regularly resolve, almost certainly by immune action, after a few months despite their malignant appearance histologically[(178)], supports this suggestion.*

The second area of interest is cervical carcinoma, of which several were reported in Starzl's survey of Denver experience[(179)]. The common occurrence of *Herpes simplex* virus Type 2 (HSV2) in this location and its suggested association with cervical cancer[(180)] raises the possibility that something not too dissimilar to the influence of EBV on lymphocytes may be taking place. There is well established evidence that early and continued sexual experience is associated with a higher incidence than in normal women and much higher than in those who have remained virgin. Infection with a variety of pathogens and semi-pathogens is usually regarded as part of the process responsible for the correlation with sexual precocity. Here again we have allperennially proliferating tissue whose activity can be modified by inflammatory conditions. As the tissue ages, there is the same accumulation of the results of somatic mutation with, eventually, the appearance of pre-malignant cells capable of being triggered to active malignancy.

There is still uncertainty about the relationship of carcinoma *in situ* to fully developed carcinoma of the cervix. The curve of incidence of diagnosed cervical cancer, most of it carcinoma *in situ*, has a ten to fifteen years earlier peak than the curve of mortality[(181)]. This is seen in most statistics and presumably means that a substantial proportion of women, who if examined would show the existence of cancer *in situ*, never develop overt cervical carcinoma. The possibility that much of what is diagnosed as carcinoma *in situ* is a premalignant stage requiring infection with HSV2 or some other inflammatory situation to trigger a cell to full malignancy does not seem to be excluded.

I have heard an interesting report of a Melbourne case of a boy of

* Sceptical pathologists have also suggested that patients under immunosuppression are much more closely watched for minor or transient skin lesions than any available set of 'controls' and that the apparent increase in frequency is not adequately demonstrated

fourteen who was troubled by a persisting herpes simplex lesion during the first year of his immunosuppression after kidney transplantation. This is a common occurrence, but in this instance a typical squamous carcinoma developed four years later. Whether the relationship of the HSV1 to the initiation of the cancer was in any sense specific is of course unknown.

One can conclude this chapter with an assessment of the part played by viruses in human cancer. My guess is that in twenty years' time it will be known to be quite unimportant. Its current popularity in the field of cancer research simply depends on the fact that there are many experimental ways of detecting viruses and their antigens. Viruses multiply, and now that cell culture has been perfected, they can be handled with gratifying precision in the laboratory. There is no need for the worker to move outside his laboratory, and with self-replicating and variable entities like cultured cells and viruses, a steady stream of complexities to investigate can be expected to provide constant interest for any ingenious scientist.

Whatever the evolutionary origin of viruses, they exist, they mutate, and they can adapt like any organism to occupy ecological niches which allow survival. In accordance with the general rule of parasitism, a virus is almost predestined to reach a mutually non-damaging relationship with its host. In the days before cell culture of viruses I spoke of HSV1 as the prototype of the successful virus producing only occasional vesicles on the lips to allow periodical liberation of virus over the lifetime of the host. Now of course we know of hundreds of viruses which in their natural hosts show no evidence of disease and which only irregularly produce disease in some artificial laboratory host.

If, as seems highly probable, some or all viruses derive from rare genetic accidents in the genome of some autonomous organism at any time over the history of evolution, varying degrees of ability to reoccupy a site in the host genome must be expected to appear with the consequences which the viral oncologists now appreciate so well. I can see no decisive evidence that viral associations with malignant disease have anything more than the most limited accidental significance in the etiology of cancer.

Outside of the laboratory the fact that a virus or part of a virus genome is present in a malignant tumour provides no advantage whatever for the survival of the virus. As far as is known, the natural history of every 'cancer virus' being worked with in the laboratory is as a trivial non-symptomatic infection transferred invisibly from one individual to another of the same species. This holds for polyoma, for SV40, for EBV and herpesviruses saimiri and ateles, and, having regard to the grossly unnatural character of poultry husbandry, probably also for the ancestral form of Marek's disease. Nature has no interest in cancer, and to speak of a cancer virus is biologically ridiculous.

We must be concerned primarily and almost exclusively with cancer as we observe it in man, and the central fact of human cancer is its association with ageing. No one has yet spoken of ageing as a virus disease, though I have heard at least one well known virologist come very close to saying so. This book is concerned with the biological nature of ageing, and if its central theme of genetic error—of chance welded to necessity—is correct, there is no more place for viruses as causes of cancer than for lice as causes of poverty.

PART 4

Other Age-associated Conditions

CHAPTER 16

HUMAN CONGENITAL ANOMALIES

'Experiments of nature'

In immunology there have been special virtues in the study of those genetic anomalies that are expressed as immunodeficiency diseases, providing what Good called experiments of nature. The division of human lymphocytes into T-cells and B-cells would not have been so readily accepted had it not been for the existence of congenital sex-linked agammaglobulinaemia, in which the B-system is non-functional, and DiGeorge's syndrome, in which the thymus is congenitally absent and the whole T-system of immunity fails.

If the system of enzymes concerned with DNA repair and replication is vital in determining lifespan, one would expect somewhere to find that infants had been born in whom abnormality in the genetically determined functioning of the same key enzymes produced frank disease and shortening of life. There is a depressing frequency of congenital human abnormalities with a major genetic component; they cover almost every conceivable deviation from normal structure and function. Many have been clearly enough defined as due to an anomaly of a particular gene resulting in an absent or malfunctioning enzyme. Another large group, however, shows more or less characteristic patterns of multiple signs and symptoms, and even if the genetic evidence points to a typical mendelian situation involving one gene only, it is often impossible to pinpoint a primary genetic lesion.

The present chapter is deliberately based on a superficial search through paediatric text books for congenital conditions of presumed genetic origin which might be relevant to our theme. Essentially I was seeking in an unfamiliar field for conditions with functional or structural anomalies of a type which on *a priori* reasoning might be associated with what I have been calling key enzyme mutations with responsibility for error in pattern replication or transfer.

In the following chapter a rather similar procedure is applied to degenerative diseases of the central nervous system in which some aspect of ageing seems to be accelerated. Most of those discussed are also of genetic origin, but it is convenient to keep this group separate from those which manifest the diagnostic abnormalities in childhood. In both groups there is usually evidence that a single gene, often an autosomal dominant with incomplete penetrance, is involved. On standard genetic reasoning this means that essentially the condition depends on the absence or malfunctioning of one enzyme.

The clinical manifestation in children of a gene lesion responsible for error-proneness in one of the key enzymes would depend on a number of factors about which virtually nothing is known. We should need to know in the first place how many distinct DNA polymerases coded for in the germ-line genome are present in the zygote, and how their fidelity is or may be modified by enzymes with which they become associated as the various somatic cell lines differentiate. Changes in the enzyme systems concerned with DNA replication within the same differentiating cell line during embryonic development could be even more important, and some of the findings to be mentioned later point strongly towards their existence. There is no lack of precedent. The reappearance of foetal antigens in malignant cells has been discussed earlier and the changes in the haemoglobin present in red cells in various stages of development are well known. Each has its characteristic structure and each must be coded in terms of specific information in the genome. On general biological principles it would seem highly likely that in the whole four-dimensional existence of a man or any other mammal there are many, perhaps hundreds, of structurally distinct DNA polymerases. We have no inkling as to what proportion of these are fully predetermined by information in the zygote; some certainly are, and all may be. In due course it will be necessary to acquire a basic understanding of the inter-relationships of the DNA polymerases in the various lines of somatic cells, including both those which continue clonal proliferation through life and those which cease replication, as post-mitotics, as soon as differentiation is complete. For any eventual understanding of the relevant genetic abnormalities it will be essential to know the stages of differentiation at which, in each cell line, one DNA polymerase (or other key enzyme) is replaced by another.

Our subject matter in this chapter is to recognize and discuss disease conditions which have an obvious genetic component but which seem to be too diverse in their manifestations to represent the primary result of a single gene change. It is well known that a single enzyme defect occurring early in embryonic life may produce abnormalities in various parts of the body without somatic mutation coming into the picture. It will be necessary to differentiate such effects from what might happen if an error-prone DNA or RNA polymerase was active only for a limited period when the embryo contained perhaps only a few thousand cells. This could result in a random distribution of mutations within the various cell lines in which it was active, including multiple mutations in lines where transcription or other key enzymes had become involved and the first steps towards error catastrophe had been taken. If this polymerase was replaced by more normal ones for the rest of development, great individual variations could be found among children suffering from a single genetic anomaly. Obviously an infinite number of variations on this theme would be possible with correspondingly various opportunities to find other hypotheses to account for the diversities.

In the light of earlier discussion certain clinical features which might be expected to be common in children damaged by a combination of genetic anomaly and overactive somatic mutation would be: progressive bone marrow failure or failure of one constituent, e.g. as shown by thrombocytopenic purpura, abnormally early appearance of malignant tumour, especially of the lymphoreticular types, multiple primary lesions in skin or elsewhere, signs of accelerated ageing, such as early greying and loss of hair.

In looking through a systematic account of patterns of human malformation, e.g. that of Smith[182], one can find a number of syndromes which, superficially at least, seem to meet such requirements.

A tentative and certainly incomplete list of conditions which fall within our limits is as follows:

A. Conditions associated with pancytopenia or other evidence of bone marrow failure:

1. Fanconi's syndrome and the probably related conditions of radial aplasia-thrombocytopenia and dyskeratosis congenita
2. Chediak–Higashi syndrome
3. Wiskott–Aldrich syndrome

B. Conditions with abnormal frequency of lymporeticular malignancy, including leukaemia.

This includes 1, 2 and 3 under A, and in addition:

4. Ataxia-telangiectasia
5. Bloom's syndrome, which has resemblances to both 1 and 4

C. Conditions showing a senile appearance at an unduly early age:

6. Progeria and Werner's syndrome

Brief accounts of some of the more extensively studied of these syndromes will be given and discussed from the point of view of their possible relationship to error-prone key enzymes.

Fanconi's syndrome and related conditions

Fanconi's syndrome(183) has as almost regular features, bone marrow failure with pancytopenia, retardation of growth, and brownish diffuse pigmentation of the skin. In addition, there is a very extensive list of disabilities that may be present in a significant proportion: mental deficiency, aplasia of the radius, ptosis, strabismus, or other eye abnormalities, congenital heart defect, osteoporosis and others.

Respiratory infections are common, and acute leukaemia may be seen; survival is seldom more than two years.

The indications are that the condition is an autosomal recessive one, but there are hints that it could be an autosomal dominant condition of low penetrance. Evidence for this depends on a 2:1 ratio of affected males to females, more than 25 per cent of siblings with the condition, and some record of parental abnormalities that might be relevant.

The only laboratory finding at the genetic level is that chromosomes of cultured lymphocytes are unduly fragile. A recent study of this phenomenon showed that the fragility was increased by DNA cross-linking agents(184). The authors suggested that this could indicate that lymphocytes in these children are defective in the repair mechanisms which normally deal with points of DNA cross-linking.

Two other conditions which appear closely related to Fanconi's syndrome are radial aplasia-thrombocytopenia and dyskeratosis congenita. The former, in addition to the two cardinal symptoms, may show anaemia beyond that due to blood loss and a variety of morphological abnormalities, including 25 per cent with congenital heart defect. One case of leukaemia is on record. The condition is regarded as autosomal recessive on very incomplete evidence. Dyskeratosis congenita is a very rare condition, thirteen cases only being reported—two females, eleven males. The signs are irregular pigmentation and other derangements of skin structure, including sometimes premature greying of the hair, premalignant leukoplakia of mucous membranes; pancytopenia develops slowly, and with malignant transformation in mucous membrane is one of the two major causes of death, which usually occurs before thirty.

The Chediak–Higashi syndrome is interpreted by Windhorst *et al.*[185] as primarily a genetic defect involving lysosomes and related cell organelles, such as leucocyte granules and the melanin granules of melanocytes. The children are very subject to infections and are prone to die of a fulminant illness with enlarged liver, spleen and lymph nodes, panycytopenia, and indications that the condition is essentially a diffuse and atypical malignant lymphoma. Light-coloured hair and diminished skin and eye pigmentation are common. Signs of central and peripheral neuropathy are mentioned. This is clearly a condition more remote from Fanconi's syndrome than the others. The evidence is good that this is an autosomal recessive, but the fact that some heterozygous parents show large inclusion in leucocytes indicates some degree of incomplete dominance.

Ataxia-telangiectasia is an autosomal recessive condition with a relatively minor growth deficiency and two major abnormalities, cerebellar dysfunction with ataxia, and a marked deficiency in T-system immunity. Presumably related to the latter is a high incidence of malignancy of the lymphoreticular system. Telangiectases (enlarged superficial venules) are seen on the bulbar conjunctiva, on the bridge of the nose, and, less commonly, elsewhere. The skin may show areas of altered hair or skin pigmentation, including *cafe-au-lait* spots. The ataxia is progressive and leads to speech difficulties, which makes the assessment of intelligence very difficult. Respiratory infections with generalized bronchiectasis are almost regular and their failure to respond to antibiotics suggests to Smith that some mucosal difficulty is also concerned. He points out certain common features with Fanconi's syndrome, both showing generalized growth deficiency, skin disorder, and a tendency to develop lymphoreticular malignancies. It is also on record that, as in Fanconi's syndrome, the lymphocytes of these patients show a high frequency of chromosome breaks in culture. Bloom's syndrome[186] lacks the cerebellar symptoms of ataxia-telangiectasia and the bone marrow failure of Fanconi's syndrome. In other respects, including chromosomal fragility, it is similar. An excess of males to females and of leukaemia in close relatives also suggests that the condition may be an autosomal dominant one with variable penetrance.

In looking over these conditions as recorded, I am impressed with the strong possibility that we are dealing with a single entity in the case of the Fanconi (radial aplasia-thrombocytopenia, dyskeratosis congenita), ataxia-telangiectasia, and Bloom syndromes, and one that may represent the activity of a 'mutator gene' at a relatively early stage. I should not exclude the possibility of including the Chediak–Higashi syndrome in the same group, but it has rather highly specific features and can be omitted for the present.

The range of conditions which for convenience we can speak of as the Fanconi group (see Table 6) all present a wide range of clinical pictures and seem to be differentiated mainly by the clinical predominance of one particular system deficiency. It seems at least as likely as any other interpretation to postulate an autosomal recessive gene with occasional partial dominance functioning as a mutator gene, presumably a gene normally controlling a DNA polymerase active in early embryonic life.

This for the present is little more than pure speculation, but if the basic concept of intrinsic mutagenesis is correct, there are two important consequences in this general area. The first is that if the hypothesis is valid we should expect to find disease conditions resulting from the activity of DNA polymerases of high error-proneness coded for by 'mutator' genes. If they did not exist, the validity of the whole concept would be in danger. The second consequence of what is in fact a working hypothesis is that it suggests that appropriate cultured cells from these conditions should be examined for evidence of ineffective repair of DNA or excess errors in copying synthetic polynucleotides. Positive results would make less likely the alternative explanation, that all the syndromes of the group derive from a single genetic deficiency, an enzyme active in embryogenesis for example, and that the diversity of manifestations is due to the other genetic characters of the individuals concerned.

The Wiskott–Aldrich syndrome

The Wiskott–Aldrich syndrome is a well defined sex-linked condition seen only in boys. The cardinal signs are thrombocytopenia, eczema (especially in infancy), and frequent infections. This is mainly an immune-deficiency disease and is discussed by Cooper *et al.*[187] from that standpoint. Most of the deficiency is in regard to the T-system and

Table 6 Five genetic conditions with multiple abnormalities

Syndrome	*Pancytopenia*	*Thrombo-cytopenia*	*Structural abnormalities*	*Dwarfism*	*Skin changes*	*Immune deficiency*	*Neurological changes*	*Malignancies*
Fanconi's	+++	+	++	+	+	++	+	+ Ly.
Radial aplasia thrombocytopenia	+	++	++	+	+	?	±	?
Dyskeratosis congenita	++	+	±	+	++	?	—	++ Ep.
Bloom's	—	—	++	+	++	?	—	++ Ly.
Ataxia telangiectasia	—	—	—	+	+	+++	+++	++ Ly.

Ly. = lymphoreticular, Ep. = epithelial malignancies. (Data from Smith[182], by courtesy of Saunders.)

this develops progressively during childhood; chronic candidiasis is common and there is a marked deficiency in tests for skin sensitization. On the humoral side there is inadequacy of antibody production against a number of antigens with polysaccharide determinants. Most of the children die in their first decade from infection, haemorrhage, or malignancy, lymphoreticular cell tumours being common, but there are many other types. At the present time there is much interest in the finding that about half the cases seem to benefit immunologically, and to some extent clinically, from treatment with preparations of Lawrence's transfer factor(188).

Here we must postulate an involvement only of the blood cell system with a specialized impact upon platelets and T-independent antibody production, plus a slower fade-out of the T-cell system. In the absence of any information about DNA repair functions in these children, the Wiskott–Aldrich syndrome does not seem to be a likely candidate for inclusion in the Fanconi group. However, the way in which the genetic character is expressed is by no means clear, and new information could change one's attitude.

Conditions of accelerated ageing

Progeria is a very rare congenital condition in which a child of eight or ten looks superficially like a 'frail, little old man or woman' and which was interpreted by Gifford(189), who gave it the name by which it is known, as accelerated ageing. There has been a tendency in recent descriptions to point out the aspects of these cases that differ sharply from the ordinary manifestations of senescence and to class it as an abnormality of growth. In view, however, of the recent finding by Epstein *et al.*(102) of gross deficiency of DNA repair by fibroblasts from a typical case, the condition becomes of critical importance for the present thesis.

Only about twenty-five cases of progeria have been reported; both males and females can be affected and there is some slender evidence that it is an autosomal recessive condition. The child is usually born apparently normal and begins to develop the characteristic facies after the first year. The principal signs are muscular hypoplasia, atrophy of the skin, and failure to grow. The children are usually within the normal range of inteligence and the brain appears to develop normally. This, combined with atypical and restricted growth of the facial bones, gives the characteristic appearance of a large, almost bald cranium over a small, wrinkled face and a beaked nose. The children are not exceptionally prone to infection and usually die in the second decade from myocardial infarction or cerebrovascular disease.

In the case of an eleven-year-old girl, described by Rosenthal *et al.*[190], who died from an accident, the outstanding findings were atherosclerotic lesions in aorta, coronary and mesenteric arteries, and the characteristic atrophic and fibrotic changes in the skin with poorly developed hair follicles. Pituitary and thyroid appeared normal. The only outstanding biochemical abnormality noted during life was a high serum concentration of lipoprotein.

Gabr *et al.*[191] described the pathological findings in a nine-year-old girl with progeria and noted that the thymus was large and lymphoid tissues moderately hyperplastic. Gifford's original case in 1904 is also said to have had an enlarged thymus.

Walford[47] raised the possibility that progeria might be a form of graft versus host disease due to maternal immunocytes, but there is no direct evidence in support of the idea, and the human examples of graft versus host disease following therapeutic attempts in immunodeficient infants have been much more acutely fatal. From every point of view it would be desirable to assess the immune system of one or more of these cases, but the reports do not suggest that any serious abnormality would be found.

Several studies have been made of the behaviour of fibroblasts from cases of progeria in cell culture, with not altogether consistent results. Danes[192] found that cultures grew much more slowly than normal and that, though there was no evident reduction in the Hayflick limit, DNA synthesis, mitotic activity, and cloning efficiency were all markedly deficient. Epstein *et al.*[102] found a limit of eleven cell generations in their case. They applied a standard experimental test for DNA repair, after X-irradiation, to cultured fibroblasts from the skin of a typical case of progeria in comparison with similar cultures from a normal donor. The DNA preparations were heavily irradiated with 10 000 R, and at intervals thereafter sedimentation analysis techniques were used to obtain the size (length) distribution of DNA units in homo-disperse preparations. Immediately after irradiation, the peak indicating average size was moved sharply to the left (smaller) with both preparations. After 30 minutes' incubation under standard conditions the normal preparation had regained its original size distribution, but virtually no evidence of repair was evident in the progeria cell preparation up to 270 minutes.

Rosenthal *et al.*[190] and Talbot[193] considered that the condition was an abnormality of growth that could not be regarded as accelerated ageing. Clearly enough it is not equivalent to a symmetrical acceleration of every aspect of normal ageing, but if, as has been suggested, normal ageing is the overall result of minor degrees of error-proneness in a number, perhaps a large number of key enzymes, this is only to be expected. If, as may be the case in progeria, the most important of those key enzymes is grossly error-prone, the result would certainly be an unbalanced acceleration of ageing, giving a picture quite unlike that seen in the average octogenarian.

If the finding of Epstein *et al.* is confirmed, as I assume it will be, these cases of progeria could well hold an important key to the understanding of the ageing process. As a working hypothesis, one might suggest that epidermal epithelium and its derivatives, fibroblasts and vascular endothelium, were subject to hyperactive infidelity of DNA repair enzymes, while the immune system and the organs whose functional cells are mainly post-mitotics were not (or much less seriously) involved. This is particularly evident in the brain, which can be of a normal weight for age; and, as would be expected, psychological testing in one case showed no senile characteristics.

These patients are particularly interesting because of the regular presence of gross atherosclerosis and excess of blood lipoproteins. Death is nearly always from some cardiac or cerebrovascular episode secondary to the atherosclerosis. If the general hypothesis is correct, this points strongly towards some process of somatic mutation being necessary to initiate the atheromatous process. Evidence for this possibility is considered in Chapter 10.

Werner's syndrome[101] is a somewhat similar condition, in which changes resembling premature senility come on at a later age than in progeria. Infancy and childhood are more or less normal, but there is failure of the adolescent growth spurt and the final height is reached at about thirteen years. The hair greys at twenty and thins progressively, cataracts often develop from twenty-five, and the appearance of old age is established between thirty and forty. Atherosclerosis, often with calcification, is regular, and adult type diabetes is seen in nearly half the cases. The mean lifespan is forty-seven and death is from malignant disease in more than 10 per cent.

Study of the growth potential of fibroblasts from a case of Werner's syndrome showed a limit of five or six cell generations for fibroblasts from skin.

Significance for ageing theory

One may summarize this account of 'a theory looking for diseases to explain' as providing to the eye of faith two groups of congenital abnormalities which would at least justify investigation along lines suggested by the hypothesis. The Fanconi syndrome group has been already discussed, with its suggestion that a phase of infidelity in DNA duplication affects a period of embryonic life. The second group includes progeria and Werner's syndrome, with Cockayne's syndrome[182], perhaps intermediate. One gains the impression from accounts of Werner's syndrome that it would be hard to find a firm line between typical examples of this and the wide range of rather unhealthy people who develop diabetes or autoimmune conditions and age early but would always be accepted within the bounds of the normal.

By hypothesis, ageing in man depends on the quantitative setting, initially by the genome, of the fidelity with which enzymes responsible for the invariant duplication of DNA achieve their objective. Significant deviation from the normal level of error-proneness will almost always be in the direction of less efficiency, i.e. greater proneness to error. One would expect, therefore, a continuous spectrum of 'genetically predetermined ages' with, as the deficiency increases and the potential lifespan shortens, an increasing number of diverse malformations and structural anomalies. One would be equally confident that many individuals with a seriously shortened potential lifespan will die from infection, trauma, or some other relatively familiar condition, without any real suggestion of an abnormality of the ageing process.

The work that has already been reported about progeria and Werner's syndrome is the prototype of the investigations which will be needed to establish the relevance of the hypothesis that these conditions are basically aberrancies of the lifespan controlling process. Current techniques, however, will have to be developed so that methods now in use for the study of bacterial genetics and of the DNA repair and replication enzymes in *E. coli* and other bacteria can be adapted to the much more complex systems of the mammalian genome. One of the first and most difficult tasks to be undertaken will be to determine the number of DNA polymerases that function in each significant type of mammalian cell and to what extent these and the other key enzymes are specific to certain cells and not others. Equally important, and probably much more difficult of experimental approach, will be the elucidation of the changes that take place in the key enzymes during embryonic development. One would certainly, for instance, have to consider the possibility that in the course of differentiation an 'error-prone gene' in a stem cell could, in the differentiated and diversified descendants, give rise to an enzyme that, as a result of changed circumstances, was much less error-prone than in the stem cell stage.

In view of the complexity of the DNA polymerase system in *E. coli*, where Kornberg's school finds four polymerases, I, II, III and III* and a non-enzymatic co-polymerase, while others call as well for 'unwinding' proteins, we can feel certain that in the mammalian cell the position is even more complex and some major methodological advances will be needed for its elucidation. It may well be necessary in the immediate future to forgo any thought of analysis of the differences between DNA polymerases at the molecular level and aim merely at refined methods of functional characterization, including error-proneness. Even that will require much more subtlety in handling cell cultures than is at present available.

Exceptional longevity

If one accepts death between 70 and 100 as the normal fate for those who avoid earlier accident, one must in principle also accept the possibility that exceptional longevity might result from an unusually error-free set of key enzymes genetically determined. According to Comfort, accurate registration of births is too recent in most countries to allow certainty that anyone has lived beyond 120. There are, however, three regions in widely separated parts of the globe, the Abkhazian Soviet Socialist Republic in the Caucasus Mountains, the Hunza valley in the Himalayas, and an Andean valley in Ecuador, where peasant peoples living at relatively high altitudes are reputed to show an exceptional proportion of healthy centenarians. The Caucasus groups have been extensively studied by Russian gerontologists, and Kipshidze[79] apparently had no difficulty in obtaining twenty-six people over 100 (the oldest 119) for biochemical studies. Death of a man reputed to be 168 was reported in 1973 in the Russian (and world) press.

In most reports the longevity is ascribed to the conventional environmental factors, freedom from exposure to infection, relatively sparse diet, mainly of vegetable origin, active manual work, and freedom from social stress. Genetic factors must play some part, and there is perhaps a hint in Kipshidze's claim that cancer and coronary heart disease are not seen in the people over eighty, on whom most attention has been directed, to raise the possibility that there are some persons with exceptionally error-free key enzymes in these groups.

Kipshidze's paper is the only one with technical data that I have found, and on loking over his tables of blood chemistry at ages from 10 to >100, two discontinuities may be seen which perhaps point to a genetically distinct population being concentrated in the 'long livers'. The results for blood cholesterol and for gammaglobulin are graphed in Figure 20 from Kipshidze's data. It will be seen that cholesterol levels rise steadily from twenty to sixty, then fall to a stable level from eighty

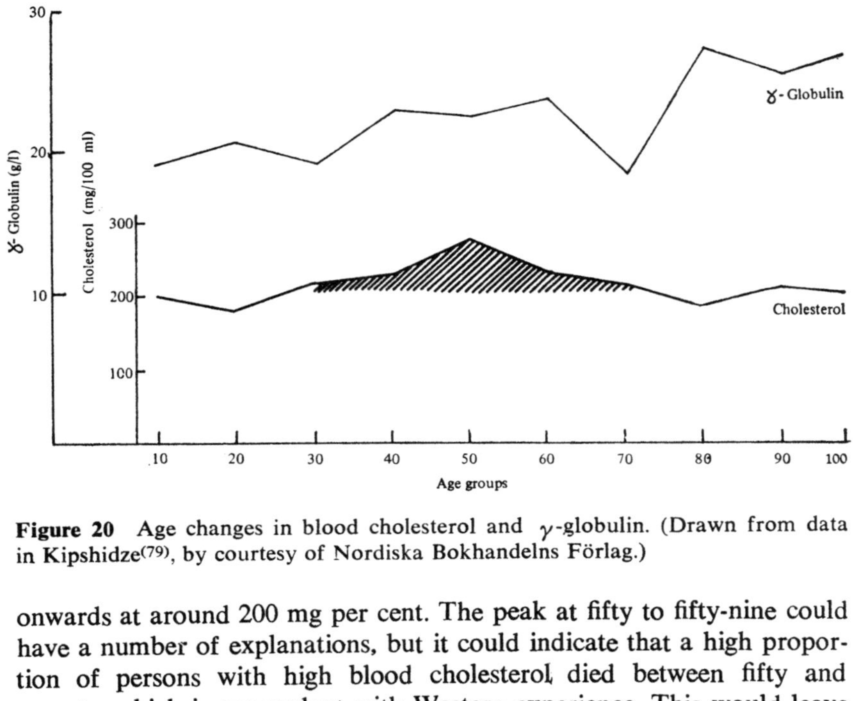

Figure 20 Age changes in blood cholesterol and γ-globulin. (Drawn from data in Kipshidze[79], by courtesy of Nordiska Bokhandelns Förlag.)

onwards at around 200 mg per cent. The peak at fifty to fifty-nine could have a number of explanations, but it could indicate that a high proportion of persons with high blood cholesterol died between fifty and seventy, which is concordant with Western experience. This would leave the long-lived group dominated by those with genetically low blood cholesterol.

Gammaglobulin figures from paper electrophoresis are also shown. Here there is a sharp dip in the values for people between seventy and eighty, followed by a high level in the older age groups. As noted earlier the gammaglobulin curve is curiously concordant with the prevalence of autoantibodies in a Western Australian country town, and suggests that the rise before seventy could represent an autoimmune process associated with earlier death, so lowering the average and allowing a later similar rise to be shown in the longer-lived moiety.

Neither explanation of these discontinuities is really convincing, but they suggest ways in which future study of such populations could clarify the positon. If a genetically definable long-lived population can be recognized, the way would be open for tests on the comparative fidelity of DNA duplication by the enzymes concerned.

CHAPTER 17

NORMAL AND PATHOLOGICAL AGEING IN THE POST-MITOTIC CELLS OF THE BRAIN

Most of our discussion of somatic mutation in relation to ageing has been concerned with clonally proliferating cells, with special attention to the cells of the immune system. A significant proportion of natural deaths can, however, be ascribed to degenerative age-associated changes in the central nervous system, where the neurones are all post-mitotic cells incapable of further replication. From our present point of view this situation is of special interest since Orgel's error-catastrophe concept was originally developed with post-mitotic cells primarily in mind with the initiation of error most probably arising at the level of transcription by RNA polymerase. It is known, however, that there is a consistent small DNA turnover in nerve cells, and one cannot exclude the likelihood that errors in the transcription process may require incidental repair of DNA with its own possibilities of error in the reconstitution of pattern.

An examination of what is on record in regard to senile dementia, and accelerated ageing with dementia as in Alzheimer's disease, on the one hand, and a number of 'degenerative' diseases of the central nervous system arising in adult life, on the other, suggests that the general concept of intrinsic mutagenesis is highly pertinent to both fields.

It is convenient to begin the discussion with those conditions where we seem to be concerned only with an acceleration and intensification of the normal process of ageing. Subsequently two well-studied conditions, both terminally associated with dementia, and with evidence of genetic etiology, will be dealt with. These are Huntington's chorea and the complex neurological disease that is very common among the Chamorro people of Guam and the other Mariana Islands in the Pacific.

Normal and accelerated ageing

Under this heading three sets of conditions call for consideration:

1. Symptoms and pathological changes in the brain in old persons who can be regarded as normally healthy.
2. Senile dementia.
3. Alzheimer's disease, which has much of the quality of senile dementia occurring at an unduly early age.

There are borderline cases, and the general tendency at a 1970 symposium on Alzheimer's disease[194] was to favour the view that, in some sense at least, these three conditions represented 'a continuum, determined perhaps by a difference in the rate of development of the relevant degenerative process'. In Roth's opinion such an interpretation would make the prospects of further enquiry more hopeful. It also offers special opportunities to apply the general theme of genetic control of somatic mutation rates to this aspect of ageing.

The most conspicuous mental symptom of old age is inefficiency of short-term memory, some degree of which is almost universal over seventy. In many healthy old persons other demonstrable changes are slight and no more than a slowing down of mental processes with a few marginal inefficiencies. In senile dementia, loss of memory dominates the early stages and develops into general mental deterioration, usually without focal symptoms. Alzheimer's disease also begins with short-term amnesia, but at an earlier age (fifty-five to seventy), and focal symptoms are liable to be superimposed on a progressive general deterioration; symptoms related to the temporal lobe and limbic area are noteworthy. Individuals with Alzheimer's disease have a strikingly higher mortality than a corresponding population of normal individuals of the same age. They represent a group, therefore, in which changes taking place in the brain determine length of lifespan. Senile dementia is a much more common condition and its incidence increases steadily with age. In a standard log-log plot of age-specific incidence, Burch[40] finds a straight line curve with the steepest slope of any human disease, 17 as compared with 4–5 for most cancers, and 11 for cancer of the prostate.

Pathological changes in the brain

The general pattern of brain pathology is similar in Alzheimer's disease (AD) and senile dementia (SD). In both, the conspicuous features are: (1) cerebral atrophy, which in AD is liable to be patchy and often concentrated on the temporal lobes; (2) neurofibrillar 'tangles'; and (3) senile plaques. The last two require some elaboration.

According to Terry and Wisniewski[195], the tangles, commonly found in the perikaryon of a neuron, are made up of twisted microtubules. They are associated with loss of neurons in the same regions and may represent a change preliminary to neuronal drop-out. Plaques and tangles are also found in close association and presumably represent results of the same general process. Early plaques, according to Polak[196], contain mostly microglial cells, but in general they are of very variable form, the most common having a core of amyloid fibres surrounded by complex accumulations of neurites and synaptic boutons, twisted tubules, and other degenerate material. 'Burnt out' plaques are simply small masses of amyloid.

In essentially normal people, plaques may be found in small numbers from the fourth or fifth decade, and are present in 70 per cent of people over seventy. Nevertheless, 20 per cent of eighty-year-olds have no plaques or tangles. There is a general correlation of numbers of plaques and tangles with the degree of dementia, irrespective of whether it is classified as AD or SD. There is no accepted interpretation of the genetic or biochemical processes responsible for the development of tangles and plaques.

Other pathological changes that may be seen in senescent brains are accumulations of lipofuscin (age pigment) and, characteristically in Alzheimer's disease, granulo-vacuolar changes in the pyramidal cells of the hippocampus. Persons who have died with SD or AD show at autopsy the expected variety of degenerative change in other organs, and, when carefully looked for, amyloid deposits are usually found. It is reported that in the last stages of AD there is often an extreme and rapid reduction in body weight.

The genetics of senile dementia and Alzheimer's disease

According to Pratt[197], senile dementia has a well marked genetic association. Kallman found concordance in 43 per cent of monozygote twins, 8 per cent of dizygote twins. The familial data are consistent with the presence of a single autosomal dominant gene carried by 12 per cent of the population and reaching 40 per cent expression by the age of ninety.

Alzheimer's disease presents a more complex situation. In the first place the sex ratio is three females to one male, and three investigations are consistent in suggesting a dominant condition with expression in only a few per cent of those carrying the potentiality. In addition, there are about a dozen families on record where AD, or some closely similar condition, was regularly transmitted as a dominant trait. There was variation in symptomatology and time of onset from family to family.

Senile dementia is very much commoner than Alzheimer's disease, so it is to be expected that a few cases of SD are found in first degree relatives of AD patients, but no cases of AD in families of SD propositi.

Interpretation of the changes

The nature of ageing in the brain is of special interest, not only from its bearing on the changes with age in memory, intelligence and other mental qualities, but also because it is well established that after early childhood all neurons are post-mitotic cells. Any interpretation of what is observed cannot therefore be concerned directly with DNA replication. This does not, however, in any way exclude the possibility of using a similar hypothesis, involving the fidelity of key enzymes concerned with synthetic processes in the cell, to account for the pattern of change which is observed.

The first point to be emphasized is the firm evidence that senile dementia is genetically determined as an autosomal dominant quality, but its symptomatic expression is steeply age-related, reaching a level of 40 per cent at ninety. Many individuals carrying the necessary genetic determinants do not live long enough for them to be expressed. The genetic situation in regard to Alzheimer's disease seems to be basically similar, but differs in the earlier development of symptoms and a considerable range of individuality in the symptomatology.

Basically the cellular pathology of both diseases and of normal old age is the same. There is a low grade destruction of neurons associated with characteristic accumulations ('tangles') of distorted microtubules in the cytoplasm. The other characteristic feature, the senile plaques, seem to be derived from damaged neurons, and the regular presence of amyloid strongly suggests that immunological reactions play a significant part in their development. The numbers of focal lesions, tangles and plaques increase with age and are closely correlated with the degree of mental deterioration and dementia.

For the development of an hypothesis of genetically determined infidelity in key enzymes applicable to ageing changes in the brain, something very like Orgel's original formulation, can be used. Any enzyme from the DNA-dependent RNA polymerase onward, whose malfunctioning can produce new errors in any protein (enzyme) synthesized in the cell, could serve as the enzyme with the genetically determined error-proneness that is primarily responsible for the accelerated ageing of neurons. Simply in view of the complexity of RNA polymerase, which in *E. coli* has a molecular weight of about 500 000 and consists of five different subunits, it is a reasonable guess that this is the enzyme concerned. It may also be wise to reserve the possibility that DNA repair is sufficiently often required in post-mitotic cells to make error by DNA polymerases important. All that is called for is some consistent degree of lack of fidelity in the enzyme complex involved in ensuring consistent production of proteins to genetically correct pattern. For convenience and brevity we can, as before, use the term 'key enzyme', or KE. By hypothesis, KE in any actual individual has a less than optimal structure, so that a determinate level of errors per nucleotide or nucleotide pair is produced. Allelic genes associated with senile dementia or Alzheimer's disease code for KE with significantly greater error-proneness than normal.

Errors being informationally at random, any build-up to error catastrophe in a cell will be slow. For the most part, cells rendered non-viable will be randomly distributed through the tissue, and a proportion of them will show morphological abnormalities before cell death and autolysis. It is clear that this corresponds very closely to what is observed. The regular relationship of the proportion of cells histologically involved with the intensity of symptoms, the clear evidence of genetic factors (autosomal dominance with low penetrance), and the steepness of the age-specific incidence curve are all consistent with the interpretation given and very difficult to explain on any simple alternative hypothesis.

Huntington's chorea

Huntington's chorea is the classic example of a well defined genetic disease in which the diagnostic symptoms usually appear late in adult life. It is an autosomal dominant condition which manifests itself by progressive development of choreic movement and ataxia, on the one hand, and psychotic behaviour, going on to dementia, on the other. The symptoms may first appear at any age between ten and sixty years, with the bulk of the patients being diagnosed in the fourth decade, the median age at onset being close to forty.

In 1972 a comprehensive symposium to mark the centenary of Huntington's first description of the disease was held, and most of my information on the genetics and pathology of the disease is drawn from the publication arising from the meeting[198]. There are several features that are of interest in the way the disease is inherited. Approximately equal numbers of males and females are affected, and as a dominant condition it can be inherited from either parent. It is, however, well established that about 80 per cent of juvenile cases with onset under twenty inherit from the father, while amongst the more usual older cases approximately twice as many inherit from the mother as from the father. The latter finding may be essentially an indication of the greater fertility of choreic women, but the excess of inheritance from the father in juvenile cases is unexplained.

In several places the view is taken that the general pattern of age of onset and pattern of symptoms is characteristic for each family group of cases and may differ significantly from what is seen in other groups. In any kindred there is a wide scatter of ages of onset and of death, with, on the average, about fourteen years between onset and death. General opinion is that, provided the individual lives long enough, there is 100 per cent expression of the syndrome in the Hh heterozygotes. There are a number of instances in which two heterozygotes have married and had children; in an isolated group in Venezuela 30 per cent of cases are said to be derived from parents who were or became choreic. It is not known, however, whether the HH homozygote shows similar symptoms to the heterozygote or invariably dies *in utero* or in infancy.

The main findings at autopsy are atrophy and loss of neurones involving, in descending order of intensity, caudate nucleus, putamen, frontal and occipital cortex. There is a marked increase of astrocytes in the same regions, many of them showing inclusions of lipofuscin.

In summary, Huntington's chorea, like Alzheimer's disease, represents an acceleration of senile dementia with focal symptoms usually playing a more prominent part. The pathological changes are generally similar and the genetic pattern of all three conditions is similarly associated with an autosomal dominant gene, but the degree of penetrance reaches 100 per cent only in Huntington's disease. None of the features presented seems to be incompatible with an etiology dependent on the undue error-proneness of a key enzyme concerned with the replication of macromolecular pattern.

Motor neurone disease and endemic amyotrophic lateral sclerosis with Parkinsonism-dementia of the Chamorro people of Micronesia

Of other degenerative neurological diseases with a fairly standard age incidence in middle life and some indication of genetic factors being important, the widespread affection amongst the Chamorro people of Guam in the western Pacific, called by Elizan *et al.*[(199)] 'the amyotrophic lateral sclerosis and Parkinsonism-dementia complex of Guam' (ALS/PD), is the one most relevant to the present discussion.

The disease is very common among the Chamorros, being estimated to cause about 15 per cent of the adult deaths and to be from 35 to 100 times more frequent than ALS in the United States. It is found almost exclusively among the Chamorros, but a few more or less similar conditions among other ethnic groups have been described from the region. Those writing on the disease leave open a rather remote possibility than an environmental agent is a necessary factor in its etiology, perhaps a virus, perhaps a toxin. There is, however, no real evidence as to its existence or nature.

Owing to the frequency of the disease it is impossible to obtain decisive evidence as to its mode of genetic transmission, but everything points to the 'interpretation that ALS/PD in Guam is probably an inherited disease transmitted through a dominant gene which, if corrected for age, is completely penetrant in males but only about 50 per cent penetrant in females' (quoted from Plato *et al.*[(200)]).

Virological studies by Gajdusek's group have failed to show any evidence of 'slow viruses', using the same methods that gave positive results with kuru and Creutzfeldt–Jakob disease. The suggestion that manganese poisoning may have been responsible has also been excluded. One feels justified, therefore, in accepting the disease as primarily of genetic origin. This does not wholly exclude the possibility that some local environmental factor is needed to allow the expression of the disease.

The evidence is clear that the complex is a unitary one. For instance, 38 per cent of the patients with initial signs of Parkinsonism and dementia subsequently showed clear evidence of ALS, while the opposite sequence was also seen in a substantial proportion. Histopathologically there are the typical findings of motor neurone disease, and cortical atrophy, with the important additional finding of fibrillary tangles and granulo-vacuolar inclusions indistinguishable from those seen in Alzheimer's disease and to a less extent in senile dementia. The latter findings were consistently found, irrespective of whether ALS or PD dominated the clinical picture. They are not found in patients dying with classical ALS or Parkinsonism.

There is a sex ratio of about 2.5 M to 1 F, and the age of onset averages fifty-six in males, fifty in females, with a wide scatter in both. About four years is needed for the steadily progressive downhill course in both sexes from onset of symptoms to death. Despite the reservations about a possible influence of environmental factors, it seems clear enough that the Chamorro disease, like Huntington's chorea, is a genetic disorder dependent on a single autosomal dominant gene whose symptomatic expression will be governed by age, and to some extent sex[(201)].

A general concept of degenerative disease of the central nervous system

In a very real sense the problem of why a dominant autosomal character delays its expression to an age between thirty and fifty is simply one facet of the whole problem of ageing. A genetic condition manifested by a prolonged latent period, followed by a progressive inactiviation and physical disappearance of neurones in many parts of the brain can hardly have any other interpretation than a cumulative development of somatic mutation involving a key enzyme or group of enzymes necessary for the faithful provision of molecular pattern. Since a single gene is clearly involved, we must find a single enzyme whose initial abnormality can in due course lead to such an accumulation of errors.

In considering the various possibilities, the first decision needed is whether the enzyme and the sequential process that its infidelity sets in train are located in the neurones themselves or in some other cell type. In line with his general approach, Burch would probably assume that the age-specific incidence of all these conditions depends on the accumulation of mutations in an immunocyte line until a suitably pathogenic clone of auto-aggressive cells emerges. Either by antibody or by direct cytotoxic action of the immunocytes the neurones are progressively eliminated by specific immune processes.

The more direct alternative, which I prefer, is that we are concerned with anomalous activity, with infidelity of pattern transfer, of key enzymes in the neurones themselves.

It has been emphasized already that even in the genetic map of phage T4 there are several loci where change inhibiting the synthesis of DNA can be located; in *E. coli* the picture is considerably more complex. Each gene presumably codes for an enzyme (protein) that plays a significant role in DNA replication. Some of them are definitely DNA polymerases, others have functions which have not yet been elucidated. Apart from the fact that enzymes responsible for the same general functions are present in mammalian cells, we are almost wholly ignorant of the situation to be expected in a human neurone. It must certainly be more complex and involve more specialized enzymes than is the case in bacteria. For each of the degenerative brain diseases that have been mentioned, and doubtless several more, one could assume that a particular one of the 'key enzymes' in the neurone groups specially concerned is genetically at fault. An abnormally high degree of error-proneness in that enzyme leads slowly to error catastrophe in the population of neurones concerned.

Choice between an autoimmune process dependent on lymphocytic mutation and an intrinsic course of error-development in the neurones will have to wait on positive experimental findings, such as the demonstration of an aberrant DNA polymerase or other key enzyme in the brain or of a lymphocytic clone with appropriately specific cytotoxic effects on the susceptible cell types.

If the hypothesis that a whole range of degenerative diseases of the central nervous system depends on the relative infidelity of pattern replication or transfer by key enzymes is eventually established, one can foresee some fascinating biochemical work in sorting out the distribution of the enzymes involved among the various functional types of neurone.

Table 7 Model of key enzyme arrangement in CNS cells

	Normal	*Senile dementia*	*ALS*	*ALS/PD*
Motor cells	A^1 B^1 C^1 D	A^1 B^1 C^1 D	$\mathbf{A}^1$ B^1 C^1 D	A^1 B^1 $\mathbf{C}^1$ D
Cortex	A^2 B^1 C^1 D	$\mathbf{A}^2$ B^1 C^1 D	A^2 B^1 C^1 D	A^2 B^1 $\mathbf{C}^1$ D
Basal ganglia	A^3 B^2 C^1 D	A^3 B^2 C^1 D	A^3 B^2 C^1 D	A^3 B^2 $\mathbf{C}^1$ D
Cerebellum	A^4 B^2 C^2 D	A^4 B^2 C^2 D	A^4 B^2 C^2 D	A^4 B^2 C^2 D

A, B, C, D each represent genetic loci concerned with 'key-enzyme' components.
A^1, A^2, A^3 etc. are alternative genes active in different cell systems.
Mutation of a gene to an unduly error-prone condition is indicated by bold type
ALS = amyotrophic lateral sclerosis
ALS/PD = complex disease of Chamorro people of Guam

Even with the limited neurological material that has been discussed, one can suggest a crude conceptual model which may indicate the possibilities. We could assume that error-proneness of pathogenic degree could be shown by any one of four types of key enzyme, A, B, C and D, each coded for by a separate set of genes. A might have a specific form, A^1, A^2, etc., for each distinct cell type, and more or less similar rules could be devised for types B, C and D. A possible situation is depicted in Table 7, which would correspond to error-proneness in C^1 having a wider and more variable effect (corresponding to the Guam disease) than in A^1, which is assumed to be responsible for amyotrophic lateral sclerosis of classical character. It need hardly be added that only when methods of defining the enzymes and assaying their error-proneness are available, could the model be used to interpret the actual clinical and pathological findings.

CHAPTER 18

SOCIAL IMPLICATIONS OF THE BIOLOGICAL APPROACH TO AGEING

The approach to an interpretation of ageing that has been developed in the preceding chapters was developed almost wholly in general biological terms. The use of human examples was mainly determined by their being much more readily available than any others. What has been almost completely omitted is any consideration of old age in the setting of the human community. In this chapter I cannot do more than look at any differences in attitudes to the human problems of ageing that acceptance of the present interpretation might call for. Perhaps a more accurate statement of the requirement is to see how accepted and currently developing attitudes to the social and clinical problems of old age conform with any novelty in my approach.

It will probably be useful, therefore, to open the chapter with a summary of what is regarded as an acceptable biological interpretation of ageing.

For every mammalian species there is a certain lifespan appropriate to its mode of living. Its length is a genetically determined characteristic which appears to be mediated approximately as follows:

1. The immediate expression of the relevant genes is in determining the degree of error-proneness of the key enzymes concerned with the replication of DNA and the accurate transfer of information to other macromolecules.

2. Any degree of error will necessarily result in the accumulation of multiple mutations in a regularly increasing proportion of somatic cells, leading eventually to error catastrophe and cell death.

3. In clonally proliferating cell lines the Hayflick limit phenomenon will usually be manifested with extinction of certain clones. It is assumed that this is of special importance for the T- and B-cells of the immune system whose progressive deterioration is responsible for a major part of the vulnerability of old age and for much age-associated disease.

4. Progressive accumulation of error in post-mitotic non-proliferating cells, such as those of the brain, can lead to loss of cells by error catastrophe and progressive failure of function. In the brain, Alzheimer's disease and senile dementia are probably of this origin and in some persons define the length of their lifespan; a number of other degenerative diseases of the central nervous system may depend on similar mechanisms.

5. Basically similar reductions of cell populations by sequential somatic mutation with error catastrophe occurs in most clonally multiplying cell lines, such as fibroblasts and skin epithelium. These give rise to some of the typical manifestations of old age, but do not directly influence lifespan.

6. Neoplasia, including benign tumours but more particularly solid malignant tumours and the leukaemias and related conditions, is the most important age-associated disease. It is also primarily a manifestation of sequential somatic mutation, whose expression may be accelerated by prolonged exposure to certain environmental agents and delayed by the process of immune surveillance.

There are only two concepts included in that outline which could have significant human implications that are not covered by any other reasonable approach to the problems. They are (i) the postulation of genetic control of somatic mutation rates and (ii) the role of the thymus and of thymus-dependent clones of immunocytes.

The implications of genetic control

According to our hypothesis, genetic control of the level of error in DNA replication in somatic cells in mediated through structural changes in one or more of the enzymes concerned in the process. To avoid circumlocution it is convenient to assume that one key enzyme is concerned and refer to it as DNA polymerase, but no significant difference would be introduced if two or more enzymes, all under specific genetic control, are concerned in the error control function. It is equally irrelevant at this level whether the key enzymes are common to many or most somatic cell types or whether, as seems likely, there is a wide range of cell line or tissue-specific DNA polymerases and other key enzymes.

Irrespective of all detail, a typical genetic process is involved and, as always, there is no way by which any practical influence on its expression can be exerted at the molecular level. The basic genetic information is in a single cell, the fertilized ovum, and is carried by a minute fraction of the cell's DNA with no hint whatever by which the actual molecules concerned could be localized. There is no conceivable way by which the pattern on those molecules could be changed to one that some all-wise geneticist-physician would consider more desirable. There are tricks by which some rather simple genetic anomalies can be corrected. If the individual lacks an enzyme normally produced by liver and kidney for use throughout the body, it is sometimes effective and justifiable to transplant a kidney from a normal donor to make good the deficiency. But there is no such approach to the 99 per cent of anomalies where the missing or defective enzyme must be present in some cell at the right place and the right time. Every genetic anomaly derives from a single cell and in nearly every case the only alternative to destroying that cell and its descendants—acceptable for a somatic genetic anomaly but not for genetic disease—is to accept the misfortune and learn to live with it. We cannot expect to use any sort of genetic engineering to increase lifespan.

In principle, selective breeding might accomplish something. Theoretically, one could extend one's prospective children's life expectancy a little by finding a spouse with four grandparents all alive and healthy, but that is a rather unreal eugenic exercise.

At the second level, the accumulation of cascading genetic error in somatic cells, going on to error catastrophe and progressive atrophy and inefficiency in vulnerable systems, also seems likely to remain perpetually unapproachable at the practical level.

However, at the stage where immunological weaknesses play a major part, there is a possibility of intervening. The function of the thymus and the effectiveness of the immune system as a whole can be influenced in several ways. If the concept of a finite 'quota of cell generations' is accepted, our objective must obviously be to make the lymphocyte–immunocyte quota last as long as possible.

Conservation of cell generation

Lymphocytes are being produced in large numbers even late in life, but they are also one of the most vulnerable of the somatic cells. For reasons that are well understood, the lymphocyte is a highly expendable cell. There is a mechanism by which hormones from the adrenal, including a form of cortisone, can cause large numbers of lymphocytes to break down and liberate their components, the building blocks of their nucleic acids and proteins, into the general metabolic pool where they can be utilized as required at the time. Almost any bodily stress can provoke that adrenal response, notably an infection. An attack of measles, for instance, is a real immunological battleground with so heavy a mortality amongst lymphocytes of the T-system that for some weeks afterwards the patient loses his capacity to give skin tests like the Mantoux test for tuberculosis, for which he was previously positive. Any other infection, any serious accident, in fact any type of disabling illness shrinks the thymus and rapidly destroys lymphocytes elsewhere.

The first rule for longer life on this basis would clearly be to avoid unnecesary illness, and in particular to prevent those diseases of childhood that can be prevented by appropriate immunization—diphtheria, measles, whooping cough, mumps, and polio. They are all diseases which everyone was liable to get in the old days, often of course in very mild form, and they can all be prevented almost with certainty by immunization. A well known gerontologist, Hardin Jones[(202)], took the point of view that senescence was essentially the accumulation of 'impairments'. He defined an impairment as resulting when any stress went beyond the physiological range of complete and rapid recovery. Most of his evidence consisted in showing that mortality in adult life was dependent on the amount of illness that each group had been exposed to during childhood. That point of view fits wholly into the approach I have been adopting.

Some classic studies on the effect of prolonged hardship on lifespan have been made on prisoners of war. There are accurate figures available for deaths in 10 000 male interned civilians in Java for 1944 and 1945. When plotted against age we still see the familiar Gompertz straight line, but it is moved, still parallel with the normal, to the left. In 1944 the curve was approximately twelve years to the left, in 1945 twenty years. In other words, a fifty-year-old internee had the chances of death of a sixty-two-year-old man in 1944 and of a seventy-year-old in 1945. A study made in America of ex-prisoners of war after release and rehabilitation showed an undue mortality in survivors in subsequent years. The trend of the figures suggested that perhaps an average of five years' lifespan would be lost as a result of the experience. Limited Australian studies[(203)] of ex-prisoners of war to 1963 gave a rather different finding. Older men showed a small but significant *advantage* over ex-servicemen

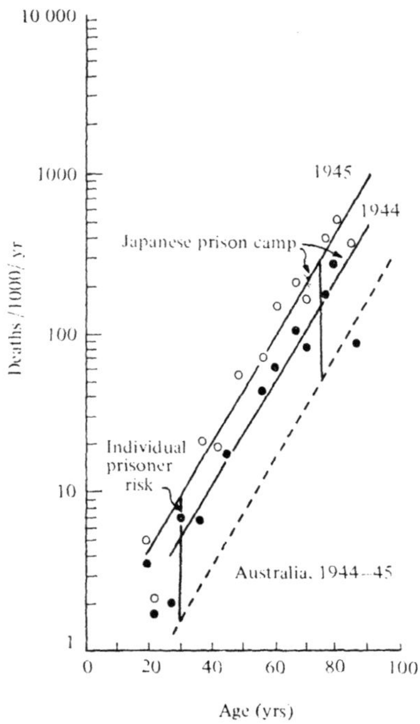

Figure 21 Deaths by age of inmates in a Japanese prisoner of war camp, ● = 1944; o = 1945, compared with similar figures for Australian civilians at the same period. (From Hardin Jones[202], courtesy of University of Chicago Press.)

who had not been prisoners that was wholly due to their better record in regard to ischaemic heart disease. Younger men showed more deaths than in the control series, with suicide and accidental death mainly responsible. Tentative conclusions, which might have to be modified when the Japanese war generation completes its term, are that the excess deaths in younger ex-prisoners had a basis in post-war psychological and social maladjustment but that older men, mostly still in their fifties in 1963, had benefited by a period of marginal malnutrition and avoided the coronary deaths of many of their contemporaries.

Some psychological aspects

It would be interesting to know whether emotional stress can play a part in causing excess lymphocyte breakdown, either in the thymus or in other repositories of T-cells; and either as a result or independently play a part in shortening lifespan. From the nature of the problem it is probably impossible to obtain a fully objective answer, but intuitively I should think it likely that any prolonged periods of anxiety, frustration and depression would have both effects. All the statistics indicate that persons in the 'upper' social classes (the professional and managerial groups) have a higher life expectation than those of lower income levels, and that those who have completed a university course live longer than those who have not. Everything that I have read or drawn from experience shows how extraordinarily difficult it is to sort out in any more detail than that what are the measurable features of a man's life experience that can help to predict his potential longevity. The intelligent well educated man with an interesting professional job is a better candidate for long life than the average, but this does not necessarily indicate that job satisfaction and freedom from money worries are responsible. It may merely be that he is more likely to apply an intellilgent moderation in the use of alcohol and tobacco and act sensibly about diet, exercise, and other things that concern his health. And, however repellent the view may be to most sociologists, there is still a possibility that most of the advantages are based on genetic differences between the groups being compared.

In all sociological investigations there are likely to be unappreciated factors which may vitiate the results. However, it is worth referring with this qualification to two studies which may be relevant. The first was commissioned by the Metropolitan Life Insurance(204) and dealt with the influence of 'success' on lifespan. The population studied covered those Americans with biographies in Who's Who for 1952—successful people who had achieved recognition in their work. A sample population from that volume was reassessed as to survival in 1967, fifteen years later, using each major category (science, literature, business, journalism, and so on). The survival experience in each group was compared by appropriate actuarial methods with figures for the overall United States experience of the corresponding professional groups as a whole. In general, these successful professionals survived better than their less distinguished colleagues, with the scientists showing the greatest advantage. The only group in which those of high achievement, as judged by a Who's Who rating, fared worse than the average of their profession were journalists.

In the other investigation a large group of over seventies, going up to the nineties plus, were examined for all the accepted indications concerned with ageing. Did they smoke cigarettes or drink excessively? Were they overweight? Did they have a high blood pressure or a high blood cholesterol? What was the age at which their parents died? Had they enjoyed their job? The various correlations gave the results one might expect, but the question that was most relevant to their survival was the last. Job satisfaction seemed to be the most important thing of all in promoting longevity.

Cancer prevention

The significance of the age-incidence of cancer has been extensively discussed from the two angles of its production by sequential somatic mutation and its partial control by immune surveillance—both intrinsic processes not obviously susceptible to any sort of clinical modification. The fact that 95 per cent of primary lung cancer is preventible and other indications of the part played by environmental factors have been mentioned earlier. From the human angle this is the most important facet of cancer and, at the risk of repeating things said in Chapter 13, we may elaborate a little in regard to the best known and most important of the environmental causes of cancer: cigarette smoking. If one examines age-specific incidence curves for deaths from lung cancer of cohorts of males born 1861–1870, 1871–1880, and so on, the conspicuous feature is that each curve is an approximate straight line with a nearly standard slope. There is, however, a fairly regular change from decade to decade as the cigarette habit spread and intensified. Each line is parallel and shifted progressively to the left, i.e. the same level of incidence is being reached at younger ages. The indications are that the process is now almost stabilized though in Australia and Britain the deaths from lung cancer will continue to rise for another twenty years until all the older cohorts fulfil their destiny.

The point to be made is that for each cohort, irrespective of the intensity of the environmental factors, the distribution over the ages has a stochastic regularity that points to an intrinsic and random process.

The next step is that it is now well established that industrial exposure to radon in underground uranium miners, or to asbestos fibres in the air in workers in that industry, produces a sharp increase in lung cancer that is virtually confined to cigarette smokers. The fact that city dwellers in Britain have a higher incidence of lung cancer than people smoking similar numbers of cigarettes in New Zealand suggests that urban smog has a similar additional effect on cigarette smokers. In none of these examples is it possible to obtain detailed age-specific incidence curves, but they are definite enough to indicate how the primary mutational process may be modified by environmental factors and how two different

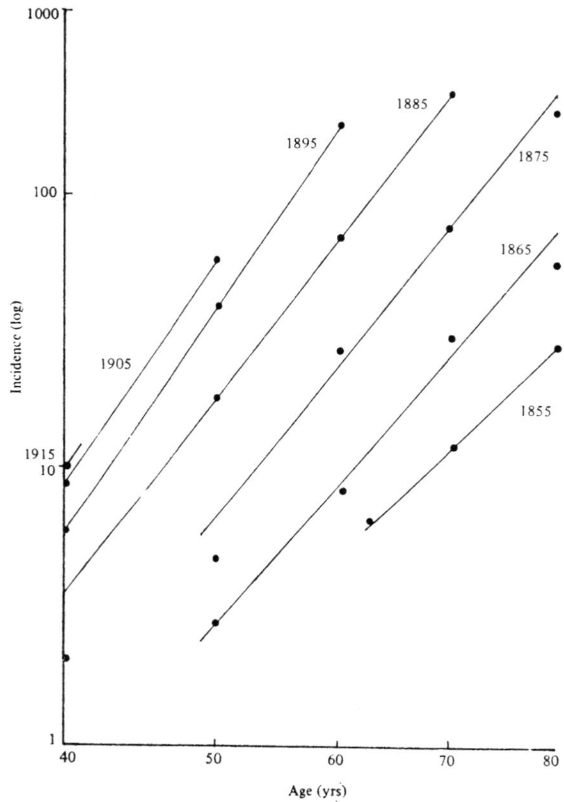

Figure 22 The changing incidence of lung cancer. The figure shows the rise in lung cancer mortality by cohorts of males born 1855 to 1905 in England and Wales. Each line shows the mortality from primary lung cancer over the period 1911 to 1955 for the cohort indicated. Note the move to a progressively younger age without much change in the slope of the curve

environmental factors can have more than a simple additive effect. New complexities may arise in the future; cigarette smoke is a very heterogeneous substance and there are already hints that the process by which tobacco leaf is matured influences the carcinogenicity of the cigarette. Some explanations were attempted in Chapter 13, but it may well emerge that the whole situation is too complex for any satisfactory interpretation at cytological or molecular levels.

From the clinical point of view, pragmatic rules for action are more important than theoretical interpretations. The only legitimate approach to the importance of environmental factors in cancer is the epidemiological one. The important indications have always been that a certain type of cancer is becoming increasingly more common, that another type is seen more frequently in one country than in another, or is concentrated on a certain range of occupations. Pleural mesothelioma in asbestos workers, the lymphosarcomas in immunodeficient patients, or the high incidence of uterine cancer in prostitutes and its virtual absence in nuns are typical examples. It is an interesting finding that to the best of my knowledge there has been only one instance where laboratory studies in animals initiated the recognition of an environmental cause of malignant disease in man. This was the fungal metabolite, aflatoxin, which has been incriminated as a likely cause for liver cancer in Africans. All the others have been identified by epidemiological studies of classical type. This will probably hold too for the still unidentified reason for a high incidence of oesophageal cancer in the region along the southern coast of the Caspian Sea or the unduly high incidence of gastric cancer in Japan as compared to other advanced countries.

The concept of cancer as essentially intrinsic to the individual is not inconsistent in any way with the recognition that environmental factors may play a major role in its clinical emergence when they exceed a certain intensity. If we are interested in prolonging the average lifespan, it is clearly wise to use every effort to reduce the impact of environmental conditions known to favour the emergence of cancer. However, it underlines my theme of the basic association of all forms of cancer with age to realize that the total elimination of cancer as a cause of death would add less than two years to the average lifespan of a typical advanced community.

What I am more concerned with is to emphasize that proven examples of environmental induction of cancer in man are all concerned with intense or prolonged exposure to the responsible agent. In my view, admittedly a minority one, every noxious agent has a threshold below which no irreversible damage is done. Life in fact could hardly have evolved unless that was true.

If this were generally accepted, many of the current mythical dangers from the environment would vanish. There is no positive evidence whatsoever that the normal level of background radiation to which we are all perpetually exposed has any damaging effect to any organism. It is only when we reach about five times the lifetime exposure to natural radiation, i.e. 25–30 R, that experimentally detectable effects are observed. In another field, DDT has been enormously valuable in dealing with malaria, typhus, and the other insect-borne diseases, and it has now been widely used for over twenty years. We have all of us minute amounts of this and other related substances in our liver fat, but again there is no evidence that those levels have done anyone any harm.

Another point that suggests a certain optimism is the phenomenon of immune surveillance. In the first fifty years of life it is highly probable that the effectiveness of immune surveillance is the most important of all the factors that can hinder the emergence of a potentially malignant cell into visible activity. Since the recognition that some tumours at least carry new antigens and are therefore potentially accessible to immune attack, various attempts have been made to devise immunological aids to the treatment of established tumours. This has nothing to do with ageing, but it does raise the posisbility that means may be developed to step up the general effectiveness of immune responses in the middle and later years of life. We have a fairly wide range of immunosuppressor drugs which damp down immunity in non-specific fashion. Non-specific potentiators of immunity are known, but we do not know whether they could safely be applied as a sort of prophylactic against cancer. One would have to be worried about unwanted and unexpected side effects, but some of these agents are already being tried in attempts to cure established cancer, and in due course a field may be found for immuno-potentiators as well as for immunosuppressors.

'Pre-death'

The hale and hearty old man or woman is no problem to society and can often be an important asset. But death comes to everyone and before death there is a period of disability and dependence. Some people have the good fortune to die within minutes or hours of the onset of the lethal episode, but for most there is a relatively prolonged period to which Isaacs of Glasgow[(205)] has given the name pre-death. He and his colleagues were studying deaths in people over sixty-five—a retrospective study to determine how long was the period of dependence before death occurred. Dependence was defined as inability to look after one's own bodily needs either because of immobility, incontinence, or mental and emotional disabilities. Dependence means that *someone must help the victim*, and here the social implications of old age come crowding in. The management of pre-death is the least attractive of all the aspects of medicine, but it is rapidly becoming the commonest requirement of general practice. Progressively the number of beds in hospitals or special geriatric institutions will need to be increased and much more research into the medical and social needs of the aged will be needed if those beds are to be used to the best advantage.

By definition there is no cure for pre-death and as yet no basic philosophy as to how it should be handled. One logical but rather melancholy finding of Isaacs' group is that the older the age at which death occurs, the longer the period of pre-death (see Table 8). In many instances, but not in all, an experienced doctor can say that such and such a patient will never look after himself again and has entered the pre-death period. All he can advise is to keep the patient as comfortable as possible and wait for him to die. Death in the old must be accepted as something that is inevitable and often desirable, and here and there one senses a distaste among the old for the increasingly successful prolongation of unwanted existence that modern medicine provides. Physical comfort, including particularly the control of pain, relief of depression by drugs, companionship, and some retention of dignity are more important than survival when the period of pre-death has been reached.

Table 8 Duration of the 'pre-death' period

Age at death	*Average duration of final illness*	
	Males	*Females*
65–74	84	85
75–84	181	183
Over 85	212	349

Data from Isaacs[205], by courtesy of *Lancet*

I believe that there is a wide scope for research on the best means of minimizing the depression and misery of pre-death in the old. Here at least is one region where the physician need have no fear of addiction just as he accepts the necessity to use increasing doses of morphia to control the pain of terminal cancer. And if the drugs needed to bring even an artificial serenity to the aged and dependent will shorten life significantly, it may be hard to say that this is a loss rather than a gain. In my opinion this is the most important area for psychopharmacological research at the present—and at the same time probably the most potentially fruitful field in geriatrics.

REFERENCES

1. MARX, J. L. (1973). Restriction enzymes: new tools for studying DNA. *Science*, **108**, 482–484
2. DEMEREC, M. and HANSON, J. (1951). Mutagenic action of manganous chloride. *Cold Spr. Harb. Symp. quant. Biol.* **16**, 215-228
3. SPRINGGATE, C. F. MILDVAN, A. S. and LOEB, L. A. (1973). Studies on the role of zinc in DNA polymerase. *Federation Proc.*, **32**, Abstract No. 1280
4. SCRUTTON, M. C., WU, C. W. and GOLDTHWAIT, D. A. (1971). The presence and possible role of zinc in RNA polymerase obtained from *Escherichia coli*. *Proc. nat. Acad. Sci. U.S.A.*, **68**, 2497–2501
5. SPEYER, J. F., KARAM, J. D. and LENNY, A. B. (1966). On the role of DNA polymerase in base selection. *Cold Spr. Harb. Symp. quant. Biol.*, **31**, 693–697
6. DRAKE, J. W. and ALLEN, E. F. (1968). Antimutagenic DNA polymerases of bacteriophage T4. *Cold Spr. Harb. Symp. quant. Biol.*, **33**, 339–344
7. De LUCIA, P. and CAIRNS, J. (1969). Isolation of an *E. coli* strain with a mutation affecting DNA polymerase. *Nature*, **224**, 1164–1168
8. CAIRNS, J. (1973). DNA synthesis. *Brit. med. Bull.*, **29**, 188–191
9. GEFTER, M. L., HIROTA, Y., KORNBERG, T., WECHSLER, J. A. and BARNOUX, C. (1971). Analysis of DNA polymerases II and III in mutants of *Escherichia coli* thermosensitive for DNA synthesis. *Proc. nat. Acad. Sci. U.S.A.*, **40**, 1064–1071
10. TREFERS, H. P., SPINELLI, V. and BELSER, N. O. (1954). A factor (or mutator gene) influencing mutation rates in *Escherichia coli*. *Proc. nat. Acad. Sci. U.S.A.*, **40**, 1064–1071
11. YANOFSKY, C. COX, E. C. and HORN, V. (1966). The unusual mutagenic specificity of an *E. coli* mutator gene. *Proc. nat. Acad. Sci. U.S.A.*, **55**, 274–281
12. SIEGEL, E. C. and BRYSON, V. (1967). Mutator gene of *Escherichia coli B*. *J. Bact.*, **94**, 38–47

13. HILL, R. F. (1972). Synergistic effect of an *Escherichia coli* mutator gene on mutagenesis by ultraviolet radiation and by alkylating agents. *Mutat. Res.*, **14**, 23–31.
14. STENT, G. S. (1971). *Molecular Genetics: An Introductory Narrative* (Freeman, San Francisco).
15. HOWARD-FLANDERS, P. (1973). DNA repair and recombination. *Brit. med. Bull.*, **29**, 226–235
16. COURT BROWN, W. M. and DOLL, R. (1957). Leukaemia and aplastic anaemia in patients irradiated for ankylosing spondylitis. *Spec. Rep. Sci. Med. Res. Coun.*, **295** (H.M.S.O., London).
17. COURT BROWN, W. M. and DOLL, R. (1965). Mortality from cancer and other causes after radiotherapy for ankylosing spondylitis. *Brit. med. J.*, **2**, 1327–1332
18. United Nations Scientific Committee on Effects of Atomic Radiation. (1972). *Ionizing Radiation: Levels and Effects, Vol. II, Effects* (United Nations, New York)
19. Nat. Acad. Sci—nat. Res. Council (1972). *Report of the Advisory Committee on the Biological Effects of Ionizing Radiations* (*BEIR*). The effects on populations of exposure to low levels of ionizing radiation (U.S. Government Printing Office)
20. ROE, F. J. C. (1973). Carcinogens and food: a broad assessment. *Proc. roy. Soc. Med.*, **66**, 23–26
21. MONOD, J. (1972). *Chance and Necessity* (English translation of *Le Hasard et La Nécessité* (Collins, London)
22. DOBZHANSKY. T. (1962). *Mankind Evolving: The Evolution of the Human Species* (Yale University Press, New Haven and London)
23. BURNET, F. M. (1959). *The Clonal Selection Theory of Acquired Immunity* (Cambridge University Press, Cambridge)
24. PUCK, T. T. (1972). *The Mammalian Cell as a Microorganism* (Holden-Day Inc., San Francisco)
25. FRASER, A. S. and SHORT, B. F. (1958). Studies of sheep mosaic for fleece type. I. Patterns and origin of mosaicism. *Austr. J. biol. Sci.*, **11**, 200–208
26. MINTZ, B. (1965). Genetic mosaicism in adult mice of quadriparental lineage. *Science*, **148**, 1232–1233
27. NICHOLLS, E. M. (1968). Genetic susceptibility and somatic mutation in the production of freckles, birthmarks, and moles. *Lancet*, **1**, 71–73
28. LINDER, D. and GARTLER, S. M. (1965). Glucose-6-phosphate dehydrogenase mosaicism: utilization as a cell marker in the study of leiomyomas. *Science*, **150**, 67–69
29. BURNET, F. M. (1972). A reassessment of the forbidden clone hypothesis of autoimmune disease. *Austr. J. exp. Biol. med. Sci.*, **50**, 1–9
30. BURNET, F. M. (1972). *Auto-immunity and Auto-immune Disease* (Medical and Technical Publishing Co. Ltd., Lancaster)
31. BENDITT, E. P. and BENDITT, J. M. (1973). Evidence for a monoclonal origin of human atherosclerotic plaques. *Proc. nat. Acad. Sci. U.S.A.*, **70**, 1753–1756
32. COMFORT, A. (1964). *Ageing—The Biology of Senescence* (Routledge and Kegan Paul, London)

33. KEOGH, E. V. and WALSH, R. J. (1965). Rate of greying of human hair. *Nature*, **207**, 877–878
34. BURCH, P. R. J. and JACKSON, D. (1966). The greying of hair and the loss of permanent teeth considered in relation to an autoimmune theory of ageing. *J. Gerontol*, **21**, 522-528
35. BILLINGHAM, R. E. and SILVERS, W. K. (1960). The melanocytes of mammals. *Quart. Rev. Biol.*, **35**, 1–40
36. STREHLER, B. L., MARK, D. D., MILDVAN, M. D. and GEE, M. V. (1959). Rate and magnitude of age-pigment accumulation in the human myocardium. *J. Gerontol.*, **14**, 430
37. SHOCK, N. W. (1960). Some of the facts of aging. In: *Aging—Some Social and Biological Aspects*, 241 (N. W. Shock, editor) (American Association for the Advancement of Science, Washington)
38. COMFORT, A. (1969). Test-battery to measure ageing-rate in man. *Lancet*, **2**, 1411–1415
39. DOLL, R. (1968). The age distribution of cancer in man. In: *Cancer and Aging* (Thule International Symposia), 15–36 (A. Engel and T. Larson, editors) (Nordiska Bokhandelns Förlag, Stockholm)
40. BURCH, P. R. J. (1968). *An Inquiry Concerning Growth, Disease and Ageing* (Oliver and Boyd, Edinburgh)
41. SIMMS, H. S. and BERG, B. N. (1957). Longevity and the onset of lesions in male rats. *Gerontologia*, **12**, 244
42. SIMMS, H. S., BERG, B. N. and DAVIES, D. F. (1959). Onset of disease and the longevity of rat and man. In: Ciba Foundation Colloquia on Ageing, Vol. 5, *The Lifespan of Animals*, 72–89 (G. E. W. Wolstenholme and M. O'Connor, editors (J. & A. Churchill, London)
43. HAYFLICK, L. (1965). The limited *in vitro* lifetime of human diploid cell strains. *Exp. Cell Res.*, **37**, 614–636
44. WILLIAMSON, A. R. and ASKONAS, B.A. (1972). Senescence of an antibody-forming cell clone. *Nature*, 238, 337–339
45. ORGEL, L. E. (1963). The maintenance of the accuracy of protein synthesis and its relevance of aging. *Proc. nat. Acad. Sci. U.S.A.*, **49**, 517–521
46. FRANKS, L. M. (1970). Cellular aspects of ageing. *Exp. Gerontol.*, **5**, 281–289
47. WALFORD, R. L. (1969). *The Immunologic Theory of Aging* (Munksgaard, Copenhagen)
48. CURTIS, H. J. (1971). Genetic factors of aging. *Adv. Genet.*, **16**, 305–324
49. MARTIN, G. M., SPRAGUE, C. A. and EPSTEIN, C. J. (1970) Replicative life-span of cultivated human cells. *Lab. Invest.*, **23**, 86–92
50. WULFF, V. J., QUASTLER, H. and SHERMAN, F. G. (1962). An hypothesis concerning RNA metabolism and aging. *Proc. nat. Acad. Sci. U.S.A.*, **48**, 1373–1375
51. BURCH, P. R. J. and BURWELL, R. G. (1965). Self and not-self: a clonal induction approach to immunology. *Quart. Rev. Biol.*, **40**, 252–279
52. CURTIS, H. J. (1966). *Biological Mechanisms of Aging* (C. C. Thomas, Springfield)
53. LINDOP, P. J. and ROTBLAT, J. (1961). Long term effects of a single whole-

body exposure of mice to ionizing radiations. I. Life shortening. *Proc. roy. Soc. B*, **154**, 332–349

54. LINDOP, P. J. ad ROTBLAT, J. (1961). Long term effects of a single whole-body exposure of mice to ionizing radiations. II. Causes of death. *Proc. roy. Soc. B*, **154**, 350–368
55. MILLER, J. F. A. P. (1961). Immunological function of the thymus. *Lancet*, **2**, 748–749
56. METCALF, D. (1966). *The Thymus: Its Role in Immune Responses, Leukaemia Development and Carcinogenesis* (Springer, Berlin, Heildelberg, New York)
57. MARCHALONIS, J. J. and CONE, R. E. (1973). Biochemical and biological characteristics of lymphocyte surface immunoglobulin. *Transplant. Rev.*, **14**, 3–49
58. METCALF, D. (1963). The autonomous behaviour of normal thymus grafts. *Austr. J. exp. Biol. med. Sci.*, **41**, 437–447
59. ANDERSON, R. E., SCALETTI, J. V. and HOWARTH, J. W. (1972) Radiation-induced life shortening in germfree mice. *Exp. Gerontol.*, **7**, 289–301
60. JEEJEEBHOY, H. F. (1971). Decreased longevity of mice following thymectomy in adult life. *Transplantation*, **12**, 525–566
61. PANTELOURIS, E. M. (1972). Thymic involution and ageing: a hypothesis. *Exp. Gerontol.*, **7**, 73–81
62. FABRIS, N., PIERPAOLI, W. and SORKIN, E. (1972). Lymphocytes, hormones and ageing. *Nature*, **240**, 557–559
63. SACHER, G. A. (1959). Relation of lifespan to brain weight and body weight in mammals. In: Ciba Foundation Colloquia on Ageing, Vol. 5, *The Life-span of Animals*, 115–141 (G. E. Wolstenholme and M. O'Connor, editors) (J. & A. Churchill, London)
64. McCAY, C. M. (1962). Chemical aspects of aging and the affect of diet upon aging. In: *Cowdry's Problems of Aging: Biological and Medical Aspects*, 139–202 (A. I. Lansing, editor) (Williams and Wilkins, Baltimore)
65. SAMUELS, L. T. (1946). The relation of the anterior pituitary hormones to nutrition. *Recent Progr. Hormone Res.*, **1**, 147
66. ASLING, C. W., WALKER, D. G., SIMPSON, M. E. LI, C. H. and EVANS, H. M. (1952). Deaths in rats submitted to hypophysectomy at an extremely early age and the survival effected by growth hormone. *Anat. Rec.*, **114**, 49–65
67. DOUGHERTY, T. F. (1962). Effect of hormones on lympatic tissue. *Physiol. Rev.*, **32**, 379–401
68. MAKINODAN, T. and PETERSON, W. J. (1964). Growth and senescence of the primary antibody-forming potential of the spleen. *J. Immunol.*, **93**, 886–896
69. METCALF, D. (1965). Delayed effect of thymectomy in adult life on immunological competence. *Nature*, **208**, 1336
70. ROWLEY, M. J., BUCHANAN, H. and MACKAY, I. R. (1968). Reciprocal change with age in antibody to extrinsic and intrinsic antigens. *Lancet*, **2**, 24–26
71. CHASE, M. W. (1966). Immunological tolerance to defined antigens and haptens: introductory remarks. *Federation Proc.*, **25**, 145–147
72. TOH., B. H., ROBERTS-THOMSON, I. C. MATHEWS, J. D., WHITTINGHAM, S. and MACKAY, I. R. (1973). Depression of cell mediated immunity in old

age and the immunopathic diseases lupus erythmatosus, chronic hepatitis and rheumatoid arthritis. *Clin. exp. Immunol.*, **14**, 193–202

73. (General reference) (1968). Birth Defects: original article series. *Immunologic Deficiency Diseases in Man* (D. Bergsma and R. A. Good, editors) (National Foundation, New York)
74. ADAMS, D. D. (1971). Present concepts in the aetiology of thyrotoxicosis. *Quart. J. surg. Sci.*, **7**, 179–187
75. CULLEN, K. J. (1972). Mass health examinations in the Busselton population, 1966 to 1970. *Med. J. Austr.*, **2**, 714–718.
76. HOOPER, B., WHITTINGHAM, S. MATHEWS, J. D., MACKAY, I. R. and CURNOW, D. H. (1972). Autoimmunity in a rural community. *Clin exp. Immunol.*, **12**, 79–87.
77. MACKAY, I. R. (1972). Ageing and immunological function in man. *Gerontologia*, **18**, 281–304
78. ACHESON, M. and JESSOP, W. J. E. (1962). Serum proteins in a population sample of males aged 65–85 years. *Gerontologia*, **6**, 195
79. KIPSHIDZE, N. N. (1968). Quantitative changes in lipid, protein and carbohydrate metabolism in relation to age. In: *Cancer and Aging* (Thule International Symposia), 49–57 (A. Engel and T. Larsson, editors) (Nordiska Bokhandelns Förlag, Stockholm)
80. RUSSELL, P. J., HICKS, J. D. and BURNET, F.M. (1966). Cyclophosphamide treatment of kidney disease in (NZB × NZW) F1 mice. *Lancet*, **1**, 1279–1284
81. NORINS, L. C. and HOLMES, M. C. (1964). Antinuclear factor in mice. *J. Immunol.*, **93**, 148–154
82. SUTHERLAND, D. E. R., ARCHER, O. K., PETERSON, R. D. A., ECKERT, E. and GOOD, R. A. (1965). Development of 'autoimmune processes' in rabbits after neonatal removal of central lymphoid tissue. *Lancet*, **1**, 130–133
83. GLENNER, G. G., TERRY, W. HARADA, M., ISERSKY, C. and PAGE, D. (1971). Amyloid fibril proteins: proof of homology with immuniglobulin light chains by sequence analyses. *Science*, **172**, 1150–1151
84. HOBBS, J. R. (1973). An ABC of amyloid. *Proc. roy. Soc. Med.*, **66**, 705–710
85. CATHCART, E. S., MULLARKEY, M. and COHEN, A. S. (1970). Amyloidosis: an expression of immunological tolerance? *Lancet*, **2**, 639–640
86. JANIGAN. D. T. and DRUET, R. L. (1968). Experimental murine amyloidosis in X-irradiated recipients of spleen homogenates or serum from sensitized donors. *Amer. J. Pathol.*, **52**, 381–390
87. WALDENSTRÖM, J. (1968). Malignancy of the haematopoietic system and aging. In: *Cancer and Aging* (Thule International Symposia), 155–163 (A. Engel and T. Larsson, editors) (Nordiska Bokhandelns Förlag, Stockholm)
88. TEILUM, F. (1968). Origin of amyloidosis from pas-positive reticulo-endothelial cells *in situ* and basic factors in pathogenesis. In: *Amyloidosis*, 37–44 (E. Mandema *et al.*, editors) (Excerpta Medica Foundation, Amsterdam)
89. BRIGGS, G. W. (1961). Amyloidosis. *Ann. int. Med.*, **55**, 943–957
90. MACKAY, I. R. and BURNETT, F. M. (1963). Autoimmune Diseases (C. C. Thomas, Springfield)
91. (General reference). 1970). *Atherosclerosis* (Proceedings of the Second

International Symposium) (R. J. Jones, editor) (Springer, Berlin, Heidelberg, New York)

92. ROSS, R. and GLOMSET, J. A. (1973). Atherosclerosis and the arterial smooth muscle cell. *Science*, **180**, 1332–1339
93. JERNE, N. K. (1971. The somatic generation of immune recognition. *Europa. J. Immunol.*, **1**, 1–9
94. VON HAHN, H. P. (1970). The regulation of protein synthesis in the ageing cell. *Exp. Gerontol.*, **5**, 323–334
95. YOSHIDA, A. (1973). Hemolytic anemia and G6PD deficiency. *Science*, **179**, 532–537
96. MCKUSICK, V. A. (1971). *Mendelian Inheritance in Man* (Johns Hopkins Press, Baltimore)
97. HOLLIDAY, R. and TARRANT, G. M. (1972). Altered enzymes in ageing human fibroblasts. *Nature*, **238**, 26–30
98. LEWIS, C. M. and TARRANT, G. M. (1972). Error theory and ageing in human diploid fibroblasts. *Nature*, **239**, 316–318
99. HOLLIDAY, R. (1969). Errors in protein synthesis and clonal senescence in fungi. *Nature*, **221**, 1224–1228
100. GOLDSTEIN, S. and SINGAL, D. P. (1972). Loss of reactivity of HL-A antigens in clonal populations of cultured human fibroblasts during aging *in vitro* *Exp. Cell Res.*, **75**, 278–282
101. EPSTEIN, C. J., MARTIN, G. M., SCHULTZ, A. L. and MOTULSKY, A. G. (1966). Werner's syndrome. *Medicine*, **45**, 177–221
102. EPSTEIN, J., WILLIAMS, J. R. and LITTLE, J. B. (1973). Deficient DNA repair in human progeroid cells. *Proc. nat. Acad. Sci. U.S.A.*, **70**, 977–981
103. KROHN, P. L. (1962). Review lectures on senescence. II. Heterochronic transplantation in the study of ageing. *Proc. roy. Soc., B.* **157**, 128–147
104. PELC, S. R. (1970). Metabolic DNA and the problem of ageing. *Exp. Gerontol.*, **5**, 217–226
105. CUTLER, R. G. (1972). Transcription of reiterated DNA sequence classes throughout the life-span of the mouse. *Adv. gerontol. Res.*, **4**, 219–321
106. KUHN, T. S. (1970). *The Structure of Scientific Revolutions*, 2nd ed. (University of Chicago Press. Chicago)
107. ARMITAGE, P. and DOLL, R. (1957). A two-stage theory of carcinogenesis in relation to the age distribution of human cancer. *Brit. J. Cancer*, **11**, 161–169
108. KNUDSON, A. G. and STRONG, L. C. (1972). Mutation and cancer: neuroblastoma and pheochromocytoma. *Amer. J. hum. Genet.*, **24**, 514–532
109. BURNET, F. M. (1957). Cancer: a biological approach. *Brit. med. J.*, **1**, 779–786, 841–847
110. TEMIN, H. M. (1971). The protovirus hypothesis: speculations on the significance of RNA-directed DNA synthesis for normal development and for carcinogenesis. *J. nat. Cancer Inst.*, **46**, No. 2, III

110a. DULBECCO, R. (1973). Cell transformation by viruses and the role of viruses in cancer. *J. gen. Microbiol.*, **79**, 7–17

111. CLEAVER, J. E. (1969). Xeroderma pigmentosum: a human disease in which an initial stage of DNA repair is defective. *Proc. nat. Acad. Sci. U.S.A.*, **63**, 428–435

112. CLEAVER, J. E. (1970). DNA repair and radiation sensitivity in human (xeroderma pigmentosum) cells. *Int. J. Radiat. Biol.*, **18**, 557–565
113. UPTON, A. C. (1961). The dose-response relation in radiation-induced cancer. *Cancer Res.*, **21**, 717–729
114. FINKEL, M.P. and BISKIS, B. O. (1968). Experimental induction of osteosarcomas. *Progr. exp. Tumor Res.*, **10**, 72–111
115. DOLL, R. (1963). Interpretations of epidemiologic data. *Cancer Res.*, **23**, 1613–1623
116. SALAMAN, M. H. and ROE, F. J. C. (1964). Cocarcinogenesis. *Brit. med. Bull.*, **20**, 139–144
117. STEWART, A. (1971). Low dose radiation cancers in man. *Adv. Cancer Res.*, **14**, 359–390
118. MACMAHON, B. (1962). Prenatal x-ray exposure and childhood cancer. *J. nat. Cancer Inst.*, **28**, 1173–1191
119. HERBST, A. L., ULFELDER, H. and POSKANZER, D. C. (1971). Adenocarcinoma of the vagina. *New Engl. J. Med.*, **284**, 878–881
120. *Transplacental carcinogenesis.* (1973). International Agency for Research on Cancer, Sci. Pub. No. 4, (L. Tomatis, U. Mohr and W. Davis, editors) cited in Lancet annotation–*Lancet*, **1**, 1425–1426
121. BOYLAND, E., (1946). Polycyclic hydrocarbons. *Brit. med. Bull.*, **20**, 121–126
122. (General reference) (1964). Mechanisms of carcinogenesis: chemical, physical and viral. *Brit. med. Bull.*, **20**
123. AMES, B. N., GURNEY, E. G., MILLER, J. A. and BARTSCH, H. (1972). Carcinogens as frameshift mutagens: metabolites and derivatives of 2-acetylaminofluorene and other aromatic amine carcinogens. *Proc. nat. Acad. Sci. U.S.A.*, **69**, 3128–3132
124. AMES, B. N., DURSTON, W. E., YAMASAKI, E. and LEE, F. D. (1973). Carcinogens are mutagens: a simple test system combining liver homogenates for activation and bacteria for detection. *Proc. nat. Acad. Sci U.S.A.*, **70**, 2281–2285
125. MILLER, E. C. and MILLER, J. A. (1971). The mutagenicity of chemical carcinogens, correlations, problems and interpretations. In: *Chemical Mutagens*, Vol. 1, 83–119 (A. Hollaender, editor) (Plenum Press, New York and London)
126. STREISINGER, G. OKADA, Y., EMRICH, J., NEWTON, J., TSUGITA, A., TERZAGHI, E. and INOUYE, M. (1966). Frameshift mutations and the genetic code. *Cold Spr. Harb. Symp. quant. Biol.*, **31**, 77–84
127. GRASSO, P. (1973). The range of carcinogenic substances in human foods and the problems of testing for them. *Proc. roy. Soc. Med.*, **66**, 26–27
128. *Demography.* Causes of Death. (Commonwealth Bureau of Census and Statistics, Australia)
129. FIALKOW, P. J. (1972). Use of genetic markers to study cellular origin and development of tumors in human females. *Adv. Cancer Res.*, **15**, 191–226
130. KNUDSON, A. G. (1971). Mutation and cancer: statistical study of retinoblastoma. *Proc. nat. Acad. Sci. U.S.A.*, **68**, 820–823
131. BURCH, P. R. J. (1965). Natural and radiation carcinogenesis in man. I. Theory of initation phase. *Proc. roy. Soc. B.*, **162**, 223–239

132. BURCH, P. R. J. (1965). Natural and radiation carcinogenesis in man. II. Natural leukaemogenesis: initiation. *Proc. roy. Soc. B*, **162**, 240–262
133. HOLLEY, R. W. (1972). A unifying hypothesis concerning the nature of malignant growth. *Proc. nat. Acad. Sci. U.S.A.*, **69**, 2840–2841
134. BERENBLUM, I. (1941). The cocarcinogenic action of croton resin. *Cancer Res.*, **1**, 44–48
134a. BERENBLUM, I. (1941). The mechanism of carcinogenesis: a study of the significance of cocarcinogenic action and related phenomena. *Cancer Res.*, **1**, 807–814
135. SMITHERS, D. W. (1960). *A Clinical Prospect of the Cancer Problem* (E. & S. Livingstone, Edinburgh and London)
136. FRANKS, L. M. and HENZELL, S. (1970). The development of 'spontaneous' neoplastic transformation *in vitro* of cells from young and old mice. *Europ. J. Cancer.*, **6**, 357–364
137. MONDAL, S., IYPE, P. T., GRIESBACH, L. M. and HEIDELBERGER, C. (1970). Antigenicity of cells derived from mouse prostate cells after malignant transformation *in vitro* by carcinogenic hydrocarbons. *Cancer Res.*, **30**, 1593–1597.
138. HADDOW, A. (1972). Molecular repair, wound healing, and carcinogenesis. *Adv. Cancer Res.*, **16**, 181–234
139. BRAND, K. G., BUOEN, L. C. and BRAND, I. (1967). Carcinogenesis from polymer implants: new aspects from chromosomal and transplantation studies during premalignancy. *J. nat. Cancer Inst.*, **39**, 663–679
140. BRAND, K. G. and BUOEN, L. C. (1968). Polymer tumorigenesis: multiple preneoplastic clones in priority order with clonal inhibition. *Proc. Soc. exp. Biol. Med.*, **128**, 1154–1158.
141. HILL, M. J., DRASAR, B. S., ARIES, V., CROWTHER, J. S., HAWKSWORTH, G. and WILLIAMS, R. E. O. (1971). Bacteria and aetiology of cancer of large bowel. *Lancet*, **1**, 95–100
142. AUERBACH, O., STOUT, A. P., HAMMOND, E. C. and GARFINKEL, L. (1962). Bronchial epithelium in former smokers. *New Engl. J. Med.*, **267**, 119–125.
143. BURNET, F. M. (1973). Cancer as somatic mutation: recent developments and prospects. *Papua New Guinea med. J.*, **16**, 3–8
144. MCKENZIE, A. (1957). *General Register Office: Studies on medical and population subjects* No. 13. Cancer statistics for England and Wales 1901–1955 (H.M.S.O., London)
145. PIKE, M. C. and DOLL, R. Quoted in Doll, R. (Reference 39)
146. BURCH, P. R. J. (1973). Smoking and cancer. *Lancet*, **1**, 939–940
147. PREHN, R. T. (1963). Function of depressed immunologic reactivity during carcinogenesis. *J. nat. Cancer Inst.*, **31**, 791–805
148. BURNET, F. M. (1970). *Immunological Surveillance* (Pergamon Press, Sydney)
149. FOLEY, E. J. (1953). Antigenic properties of methylcholanthrene-induced tumors in mice of the strain of origin. *Cancer Res.*, **13**, 835–837
150. KLEIN, G. (1966). Tumor antigens. *Ann. Rev. Microbiol.*, **20**, 223–252
151. KLEIN, G., SJÖGREN, H. O., KLEIN, E. and HELLSTRÖM, K. E. (1960). Demonstration of resistance against methylcholanthrene-induced sarcomas in the primary autochthonous host. *Cancer Res.*, **20**, 1561–1572

152. BURNET, F. M. (1971). *Genes, Dreams and Realities* (Medical and Technical Publishing Co. Ltd., Lancaster)
153. BALDWIN, R. W., GLAVES, D. and PIMM, M. V. (1971). Embryonic and tumour antigens. *Lancet*, **2**, 767
154. PREHN, R. T. (1969). The relationship of immunology to carcinogenesis. *Ann. N.Y. Acad. Sci.*, **164**, 449–457
155. KLEIN, G. (in press). The Epstein-Barr virus (EBV). In: *The Herpes Viruses* (A. Kaplan, editor) (Academic Press, New York and London)
156. STEIN, H., LENNERT, K. and PARWARESCH, M. R. (1972). Malignant lymphomas of B-cell type. *Lancet*, **2**, 855–857
157. WALDMAN, T. A., STROBER, W. and BLAESE, R. M. (1972). N.I.H. Conference. Immunodeficiency disease and malignancy. *Ann. int. Med.*, **77**, 605–628
158. HOOVER, R. and FRAUMENI, J. F. (1973). Risk of cancer in renal-transplant recipients. *Lancet*, **2**, 55–57
159. BURNET, F. M. (in press). Transfer factor—a theoretical discussion. *J. Allergy clin. Immunol.*
160. JERNE, N. K. (1973). The immune system. *Scientific American*, **52**, 65
161. KLEIN, G. (1971). Immunological aspects of Burkitt's lymphoma. *Adv. Immunol.*, **14**, 187–250
162. KLEIN, G. (in press). Epstein–Barr virus (EBV)-induced transformation of human lymphoid cells and immunosurveillance against lymphoma development. *Ann. d'immunologie*
163. KLEIN, G. (in press), Immunological surveillance against tumors. In: *Annual Symposium of Tumor Immunology*, (R. W. Cuhley and M. Abbott, editors) (University of Texas, Austin)
164. FIALKOW, P. J., KLEIN, G., GARTLER, S. M. and CLIFFORD, P. (1970). Clonal origin for individual Burkitt tumours. *Lancet*, **1**, 384–386
165. BURKITT, D. (1969). Etiology of Burkitt's lymphoma—an alternative hypothesis to a vectored virus. *J. nat. Cancer Inst.*, **42**, 19–28
166. COREA, P. and O'CONOR, G. T. (1973). Geographic pathology of lymphoreticular tumors. *J. nat. Cancer Inst.*, **50**, 1609–1618
167. COLE, P. (1972). Epidemiology of Hodgkin's disease. *J. Amer. med. Assoc.*, **222**, 1636–1639
168. GOLDMAN, J. M. and AISENBERG, A. C. (1970). Incidence of antibody to EB virus, herpes simplex, and cytomegalovirus in Hodgkin's disease. *Cancer*, **26**, 327–331
169. LUKES, R. J., TINDLE, B. H. and PARKER, J. W. (1969). Reed-Sternberg-like cells in infectious mononucleosis. *Lancet*, **2**, 1003–1004
170. WRIGHT, D. H. (1970). Reed-Sternberg-like cells in recurrent Burkitt lymphomas. *Lancet*, **1**, 1052–1053
171. KLEMOLA, E. and KÄÄRIÄINEN, L. (1965). Cytomegalovirus as a possible cause of a disease resembling infectious mononucleosis. *Brit. med. J.*, **2**, 1099–1102
171a. KLEMOLA, E., VON ESSEN, R., HENLE, G. and HENLE, W. (1970). Infectious-mononucleosis-like disease with negative heterophil agglutination test. Clinical features in relation to Epstein–Barr virus and cytomegalovirus antibodies. *J. infect. Dis.*, **121**, 608–614
172. SIIM, J. C. (1952). Studies on acquired toxoplasmosis. II. Report of a case

with pathological changes in a lymph node removed at biopsy. *Acta path. microbiol. scand.*, **30**, 104–108.
173. KELLY, W. D. and GOOD, R. A. (1968). Immunologic deficiency in Hodgkin's disease. In: *Birth Defects—Immunologic Deficiency Diseases in Man*, 349–354 (D. Bergsma and R. A. Good, editors) (National Foundation, New York)
174. AISENBERG, A. C. (1962). Studies on delayed hypersensitivity in Hodgkin's disease. *J. clin. Invest.*, **41**, 1964–1970
175. BURNET, F. M. (1968). Measles as an index of immunological function. *Lancet*, **2**, 610–613
176. WALDER, B. K., ROBERTSON, M. R. and JEREMY, D. (1971). Skin cancer and immunosuppression. *Lancet*, **2**, 1282–1283
177. MARSHALL, V. (in press). Pre-malignant and malignant skin tumours in immuno-suppressed patients. *Transplantation*
178. BROWN, F. C. and TAN, E. M. (1973). Immunological reaction in kerato-acanthoma, a spontaneously resolving skin tumor. *Cancer Res.*, **33**, 2030–2033
179. STARZL, T. E., PENN, I., PUTNAM, C. W., GROTH, C. G. and HALGRIMSON, C. G. (1971). Iatrogenic alterations of immunologic surveillance in man and their influence or malignancy. *Transplant. Rev.*, **7**, 112–145
180. SPRECHER-GOLDBERGER, S., THIRY, L., CATTOOR, J. P., R. HOOGHE and PESTIAU, J. (1970). Herpesvirus type 2 infection and carcinoma of the cervix. *Lancet*, **2**, 266
181. LEJSSNER, H. and NYSTRÖM, C. (1968). Cancer of the cervix uteri—and aging. In: *Cancer and Aging* (Thule International Symposia), 183–199 (A. Engel and T. Larsson, editors) (Nordiska Bokhandelns Förlag, Stockholm)
182. SMITH, D. W. (1970). *Recognizable Patterns of Human Malformation: Genetic, Embryologic, and Clinical Aspects* (Saunders, Philadelphia)
183. FANCONI, G. (1964). Die familiäre Panmyelopathie. *Schweiz, med. Wschr.*, **94**, 1309–1318
184. SASAKI, M. S. and TONOMORA, A. (1973). A high susceptibility of Fanconi's anaemia to chromosome breakage by DNA cross linking agents. *Cancer Res.*, **33**, 1829–1836
185. WINDHORST, D. B., WHITE, J. G., DENT, P. B., DECKER, J. and GOOD, R. A. (1968). Defective defense associated with genetic disease of subcellular organelles. In: *Birth Defects—Immunologic Deficiency Diseases in Man*, 424–432 (D. Bergsman and R. A. Good, editors) (National Foundation, New York)
186. BLOOM, D. (1966). The syndrome of congenital telangiectatic erythema and stunted growth. *J. Pediat.*, **68**, 103–113
187. COOPER, M. D., CHASE, H. P., LOWMAN, J. T., KRIVIT, W. and GOOD, R. A. (1968). Wiskott-Aldrich syndrome. *Amer. J. Med.*, **44**, 499–513
188. SPITLER, L. E., LEVIN, A. S., STITES, D. P., FUDENBERG, H. H., PIROFSKY, B., AUGUST, C. S., STEIHM, E. R., HITZIG, W. H. and GATTI, R. A. (1972). The Wiskott–Aldrich syndrome—results of transfer factor therapy. *J. clin. Invest.*, **51**, 3216–3224
189. GIFFORD, H. (1904). Progeria: a form of senilism. *Practitioner*, **73**, 188–217

190. ROSENTHAL, I. M., BRONSTEIN, I. P., ALLENBACH, F. D., PRUZANSKY, S. and ROSENWALD, A. K. (1956). Progeria. *Pediatrics*, **18**, 565–577
191. GABR, M., HASHEM, N., HASHEM, M., FAHMI, A. and SAFOUH, M. (1960). Progeria, a pathologic study. *J. Pediat.*, **57**, 70–77
192. DANES, B. S. (1971). Progeria: a cell culture study on aging. *J. clin. Invest.*, **50**, 2000–2003
193. TALBOT, N. B., BUTLER, A. M., PRATT, E. L., MACLACHLAN, E. A. and TANNHEIMER, J. (1945). Progeria: clinical, metabolic and pathologic studies on a patient. *Amer. J. Dis. Child.*, **69**, 267–279
194. (General reference) (1970). *Alzheimer's Disease and Related Conditions* (Ciba Foundation Symposium) (G. E. W. Wolstenholme and M. O'Connor, editors) (J. & A. Churchill, London)
195. TERRY, R. D. and WISNIEWSKI, H. (1970). The ultrastructure of the neurofibrillary tangle and the senile plaque. In: *Alzheimer's Disease and Related Conditions* (Ciba Foundation Symposium), 145–164 (G. E. W. Wolstenholme and M. O'Connor, editors) (J. & A. Churchill, London)
196. POLAK, M. (1970). In: *Alzheimer's Disease and Related Conditions* (Ciba Foundation Symposium), 129 (G. E. W. Wolstenholme and M. O'Connor, editors) (J. & A. Churchill, London)
197. PRATT, R. T. C. (1970). The genetics of Alzheimer's disease. In: *Alzheimer's Disease and Related Conditions* (Ciba Foundation Symposium), 137–139 (G. E. W. Wolstenholme and M. O'Connor, editors) (J. & A. Churchill, London)
198. PAULSON, G. and ALLEN, N. (1970). Huntington's chorea. In: *Genetic Disorders of Man*, 547–548 (R. M. Goodman, editor) (Little, Brown, Boston)
199. ELIZAN, T. S., HIRANO, A., ABRAMS, B. M., NEED, R. L., VAN NUIS, C. and KURLAND, L. T. (1966). Amyotrophic lateral sclerosis and Parkinsonism–dementia complex of Guam. *Arch. Neurol.*, **14**, 356–368
200. PLATO, C. C., CRUZ, M. T. and KURLAND, L. T. (1969). Amyotrophic lateral sclerosis and Parkinsonism–dementia complex of Guam: further gentic investigations. *Amer, J. hum. Genet.*, **21**, 133–141
201. PLATO, C. C., REED, D. M., ELIZAN, T. S. and KURLAND, L. T. (1967). Amyotrophic lateral sclerosis/Parkinsonism–dementia complex of Guam. IV. Familial and genetic investigations. *Amer. J. hum. Genet.*, **91**, 617–632
202. JONES, H. B. (1959). The relation of human health to age, place and time. In: *Handbook of Ageing and the Individual*, 336–363 (J. E. Birren, editor) (University of Chicago Press, Chicago)
203. FREED, G. and STRINGER, P. B. (1968). Comparative mortality experience 1946–1963 among former Australian prisoners of war of the Japanese. *Repatriation Department, Commonwealth of Australia, Medical Research Bulletin No. 2*
204. *Metropolitan Life Insurance Company Statistical Bulletin 49* (January 1968) Longevity of prominent men. Who's Who study.
205. ISAACS, B., MCKECHAN, A., GUNN, J., MCMILLAN, I. and NEVILLE, Y. (1971). The concept of pre-death. *Lancet*, **1**, 1115–1118

INDEX

GPSR Compliance

The European Union's (EU) General Product Safety Regulation (GPSR) is a set of rules that requires consumer products to be safe and our obligations to ensure this.

If you have any concerns about our products, you can contact us on ProductSafety@springernature.com

In case Publisher is established outside the EU, the EU authorized representative is:

Springer Nature Customer Service Center GmbH
Europaplatz 3
69115 Heidelberg, Germany

Batch number: 10607212

Printed by Printforce, the Netherlands